THE NURSE'S ANATOMY AND PHYSIOLOGY COLOURING BOOK

Sara Miller McCune founded SAGE Publishing in 1965 to support the dissemination of usable knowledge and educate a global community. SAGE publishes more than 1000 journals and over 800 new books each year, spanning a wide range of subject areas. Our growing selection of library products includes archives, data, case studies and video. SAGE remains majority owned by our founder and after her lifetime will become owned by a charitable trust that secures the company's continued independence.

Los Angeles | London | New Delhi | Singapore | Washington DC | Melbourne

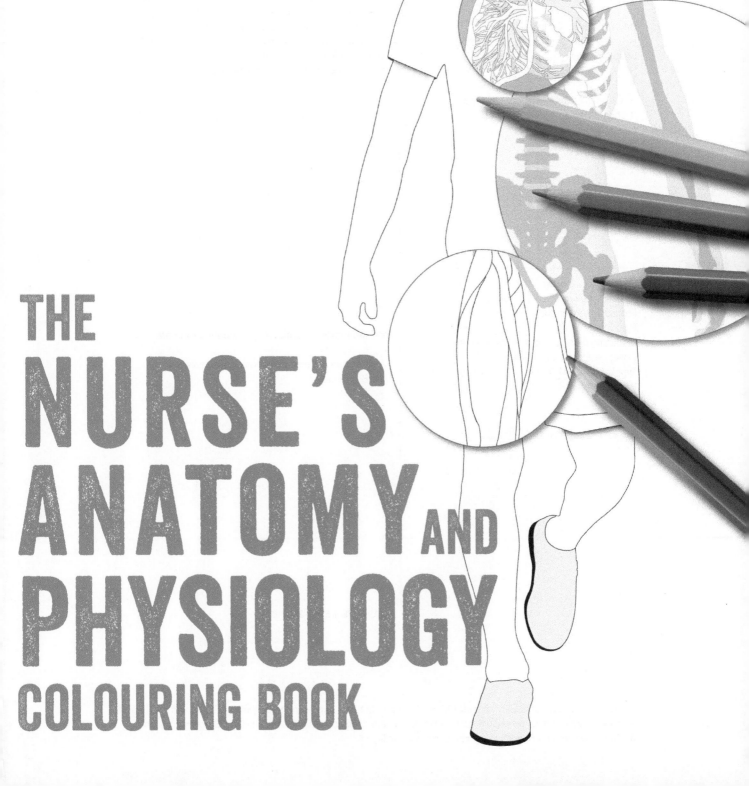

JENNIFER BOORE
NEAL COOK
ANDREA SHEPHERD

THE NURSE'S ANATOMY AND PHYSIOLOGY COLOURING BOOK

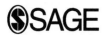

Los Angeles | London | New Delhi
Singapore | Washington DC | Melbourne

SAGE Publications Ltd
1 Oliver's Yard
55 City Road
London EC1Y 1SP

SAGE Publications Inc.
2455 Teller Road
Thousand Oaks, California 91320

SAGE Publications India Pvt Ltd
B 1/I 1 Mohan Cooperative Industrial Area
Mathura Road
New Delhi 110 044

SAGE Publications Asia-Pacific Pte Ltd
3 Church Street
#10-04 Samsung Hub
Singapore 049483

Editor: Alex Clabburn
Assistant editor: Charlène Burin
Production editor: Katie Forsythe
Proofreader: Andy Baxter
Marketing manager: Tamara Navaratnam
Cover design: Shaun Mercier
Typeset by: C&M Digitals (P) Ltd, Chennai, India
Printed in the UK

British Library Cataloguing in Publication data

A catalogue record for this book is available from
the British Library

ISBN 978-1-5264-2435-8

At SAGE we take sustainability seriously. Most of our products are printed in the UK using FSC papers and boards.
When we print overseas we ensure sustainable papers are used as measured by the PREPS grading system.
We undertake an annual audit to monitor our sustainability.

TABLE OF CONTENTS

ABOUT THE AUTHORS

Professor Jennifer Boore is Emeritus Professor of Nursing at the School of Nursing, Ulster University. Jenny started her career as a registered nurse, followed by becoming a midwife. She practised as a nurse and midwife in the UK and Australia for some years before returning and beginning her first degree in human biology. After working as a clinical teacher with the degree students she obtained a Research Fellowship at the University of Manchester and completed her PhD on pre-operative preparation of patients. From 1977 to 1984 Jenny worked as a Lecturer in Nursing at the Universities of Edinburgh and Hull and was then appointed as Professor of Nursing at the University of Ulster in 1984 (the first Professor of Nursing in Ireland). Jenny has an extensive background in education, research and professional regulation. She has taught anatomy, physiology and pathophysiology to undergraduate and post-graduate nursing students across a number of courses throughout her career. Her contributions to nursing have been recognised in achieving the honours of Fellow of the Royal College of Nursing in 1993 and Officer of the Order of the British Empire in 1996. Jenny continues to be active in nursing education and research.

Dr Neal Cook is a Reader at the School of Nursing, Ulster University and a Fellow of the Higher Education Academy. He is also President of the European Association of Neuroscience Nurses and an Executive Board Member of the British Association of Neuroscience Nurses. Neal has taught anatomy, physiology and pathophysiology to undergraduate and post-graduate nursing students across a number of courses since he commenced working in higher education. Neal is also an Advanced Life Support Instructor, teaching life support courses in Health and Social Care Trusts and in the University. He has worked in the fields of neurosciences and critical care since registering as a nurse, becoming a specialist practitioner and subsequently moving into education and research. Neal has published clinical, research and education papers in the fields of education and neurosciences and remains very active in these endeavours. He remains clinically active in neurosciences and remains a Registered Nurse with the Nursing and Midwifery Council (UK).

Andrea Shepherd is a Lecturer in Nursing at the School of Nursing, Ulster University and a Fellow of the Higher Education Academy. She has taught anatomy, physiology and pathophysiology to undergraduate nursing students across a number of courses since she commenced working in higher education. Andrea is also an Advanced Life Support Instructor, teaching life support courses in Health and Social Care Trusts and in the University. She has worked in the fields of critical care and orthopaedics since registering as a nurse, becoming a specialist practitioner and subsequently moving into education. She currently takes a lead role in adult pre-registration nursing, is clinically active in critical care and remains a Registered Nurse with the Nursing and Midwifery Council (UK).

The School of Nursing at Ulster provides pre-registration and post-registration nursing education across two campuses in Northern Ireland and internationally. The Person-Centred Nursing Framework (McCormack and McCance, 2010) is currently the curricular framework for pre-registration nursing courses at the School and influences a wide variety of programmes and research activity within the School and the Institute of Nursing and Health Research. Both the School and the Institute of Nursing and Health Research are recognised as excellent and leading in their field nationally and internationally.

McCormack, B. and McCance, T. (2010) *Person-centred Nursing: Theory and Practice*. Oxford: Wiley-Blackwell.

How to use this book

'Mere colour, unspoiled by meaning, and unallied with definite form, can speak to the soul in a thousand different ways.'

OSCAR WILDE

'Why do two colors, put one next to the other, sing? Can one really explain this?'

PABLO PICASSO

'The beauty and mystery of this world only emerges through affection, attention, interest and compassion... open your eyes wide and actually see this world by attending to its colors, details and irony.'

ORHAN PAMUK

Colours can have deep psychological effects on our perceptions and feelings. Colour grabs our attention and can arouse our emotions in distinctive and unique ways. Colour also interacts with our memory and can improve our ability to recall information. Combine this with the act of physically putting pencil to paper and you have one of the most effective ways of studying anatomy and physiology. Colouring helps you to engage with structural detail in a deeper way, making it easier to retain knowledge and make connections. It can also be fun, relaxing and an effective alternative to detailed reading.

Revise key topics with short introductions

Follow the colouring notes through each activity

Add labels to test your knowledge

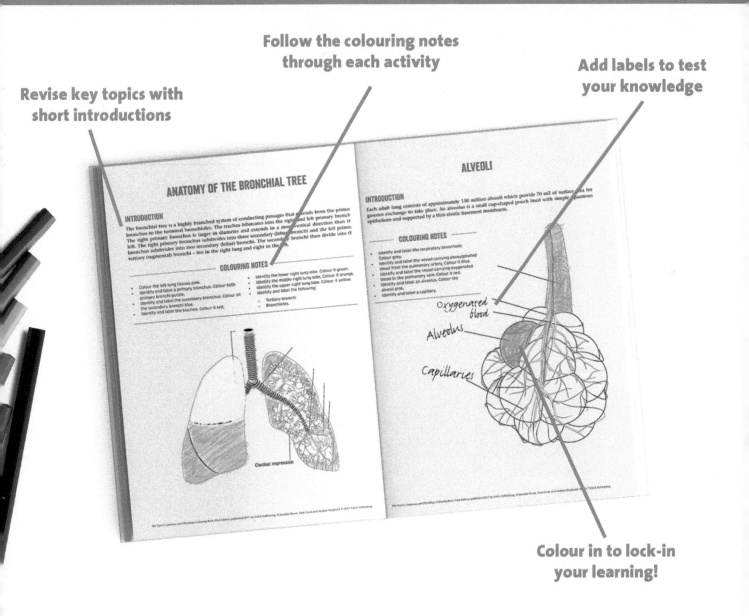

Colour in to lock-in your learning!

You will need several different colours to get the most from the exercises:

- Black
- Blue (light and dark shades)
- Brown (light and dark shades)
- Green (light and dark shades)
- Grey
- Magenta

- Orange
- Pink
- Purple
- Red
- Yellow

Most 24 packs of colouring pencils will have these colours available within them.

We hope you enjoy using this book and find it helpful as you continue to develop your knowledge of anatomy and physiology. **Good luck!**

ACKNOWLEDGEMENTS

The authors would like to thank their family, friends and colleagues for their ongoing support and encouragement while we have developed this book. This is very much appreciated and is central to bringing such projects to fruition. We would also like to acknowledge the team at Sage for their support, feedback and enthusiasm for the book; it is always a pleasure to work with you.

PUBLISHER'S ACKNOWLEDGEMENTS

The publishers would like to thank the following individuals for their invaluable feedback on the proposal of the book:

John Alcock, Bangor University, UK

Debbie King, Canterbury Christ Church University, UK

Felicity Page, University of Wales Trinity Saint David, UK

Anne Williams, Queen Margaret University, UK

CHAPTER 1

DESCRIPTORS OF THE BODY

INTRODUCTION

In learning about the anatomy and physiology of the people for whom you will be caring, you also need to understand the different terms used to identify positions and movements of the different parts of the body. This chapter will help you review some of the relevant terms. Remember to revise Appendix 3 in *Essentials of Anatomy and Physiology for Nursing Practice*.

Answers to the labelling exercises can be found at the back of the book.

ANATOMICAL NAMES

INTRODUCTION

The anatomical position is the upright stance of the body with the face forward, the arms at the side, and the palms of the hands facing forward. It is used when describing the relation of body parts to one another.

COLOURING NOTES 1.1

- ☐ Identify and label the left shoulder. Shade it red.
- ☐ Identify and label the left lower leg. Shade it purple.
- ☐ Identify and label the left forearm. Shade it blue.
- ☐ Identify and label the left arm. Shade it green.
- ☐ Identify and label the left hand. Shade it pink.
- ☐ Identify and label the left thigh. Shade it yellow.
- ☐ Identify and label the chest. Shade it orange.

- ☐ Identify and label the abdomen. Shade it pink.
- ☐ Identify and label the following:
  - ○ Knee
  - ○ Hip
  - ○ Heel
  - ○ Cubital fossa
  - ○ Wrist
  - ○ Foot
  - ○ Umbilicus
  - ○ Palm.

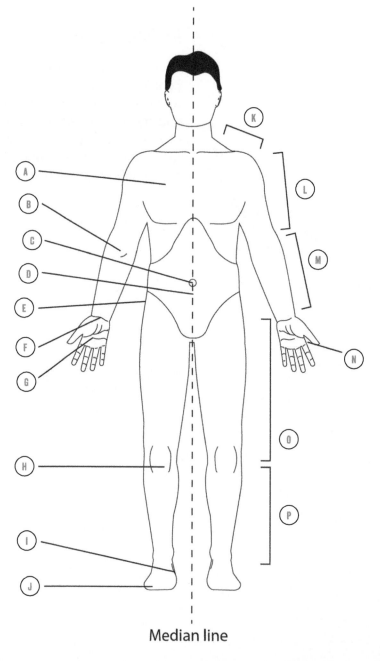

Median line

COLOURING NOTES 1.2

☐   Identify and label the left shoulder. Shade both shoulders red.
☐   Identify and label the left elbow. Shade both elbows purple.
☐   Identify and label the loin. Shade it blue.
☐   Identify and label the left buttock. Shade both buttocks green.
☐   Identify and label the left popliteal fossa. Shade both pink.
☐   Identify and label the left thigh. Shade both thighs yellow.
☐   Identify and label the left ankle and heel. Shade both orange.
☐   Identify and label the left calf. Shade both calves purple.

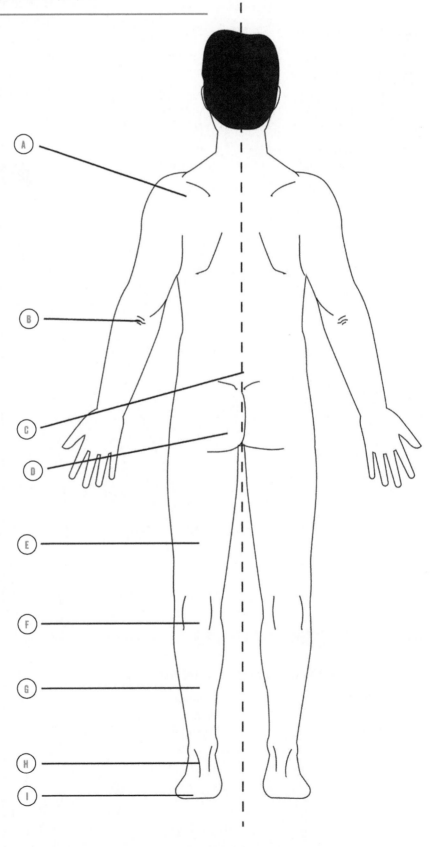

ANATOMICAL DIRECTIONS

INTRODUCTION

The table below shows the terms used to indicate the relative positions of the organs and parts of the body.

Ventral/ anterior	Front of the body	Dorsal/ posterior	Back of the body
Superior	Above	Inferior	Below
Medial	Towards the midline	Lateral	Away from the midline
Proximal	Closer to point of origin or body	Distal	Further from point of origin or body
Superficial	Closer to body surface	Deep	Further from body surface

The body can be divided by three lines:
- Horizontal: into superior (upper/above) and inferior (lower/below).
- Sagittal: into right and left halves either side of the median line.
- Coronal: into anterior (front half) and posterior (back half).

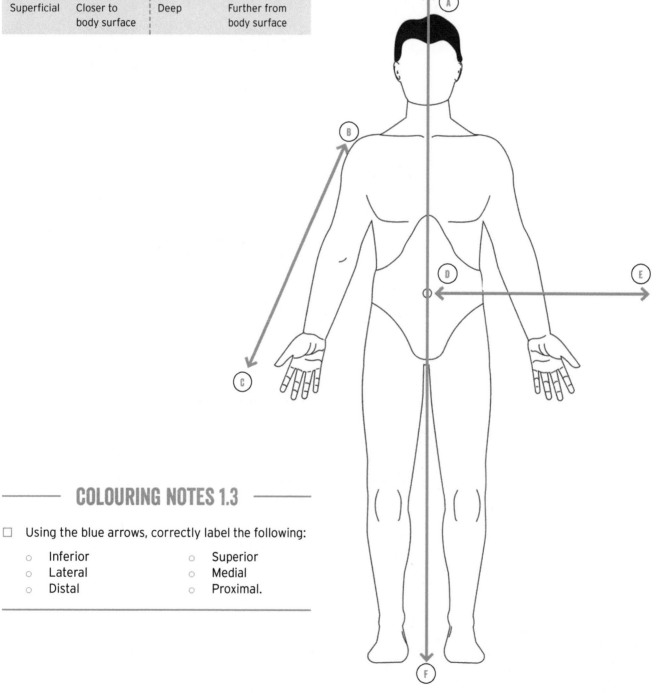

—— COLOURING NOTES 1.3 ——

☐ Using the blue arrows, correctly label the following:

- ○ Inferior
- ○ Lateral
- ○ Distal
- ○ Superior
- ○ Medial
- ○ Proximal.

THE QUADRANTS AND REGIONS OF THE ABDOMEN

INTRODUCTION

The sections of the abdomen can be divided into four quadrants or nine regions. These are used to describe location, for example the site of pain being described by someone.

--- **COLOURING NOTES 1.4** ---

☐ Identify the left lumbar region. Shade it grey.
☐ Identify the umbilical region. Shade it light brown.
☐ Identify the right upper quadrant. Shade it red.
☐ Identify the left upper quadrant. Shade it yellow.
☐ Identify the left hypochondriac region. Shade it orange.
☐ Identify the right lumbar region. Shade it pink.
☐ Identify the left iliac region. Shade it purple.
☐ Identify the right iliac region. Shade it dark blue.

☐ Identify the right hypochondriac region. Shade it dark green.
☐ Identify the right lower quadrant. Shade it light green.
☐ Identify the left lower quadrant. Shade it light blue.
☐ Identify the epigastric region. Shade it dark brown.
☐ Identify the hypogastric region. Shade it magenta.

See p. 555 of *Essentials of Anatomy and Physiology for Nursing Practice* to check the answers.

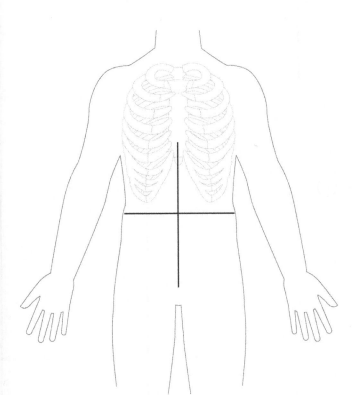

The four abdominal quadrants

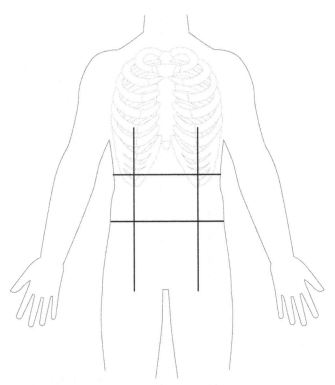

The nine regions of the abdominal cavity

BODY CAVITIES AND SUBDIVISIONS

INTRODUCTION

Anatomical structures are often designated in terms of the cavity in which they are located. Membranes, sheaths and other structures enable internal organisation of body structures by separating them into compartments. The internal organs of the body are distributed through two main cavities, dorsal (posterior/ back) and ventral (anterior/front) with subdivisions.

COLOURING NOTES 1.5

- ☐ Identify and label the following:
  - ○ Ventral cavity
  - ○ Diaphragm
  - ○ Dorsal cavity
  - ○ Abdominopelvic cavity.
- ☐ Identify and label the pelvic cavity. Colour it yellow.

- ☐ Identify and label the thoracic cavity. Colour it blue.
- ☐ Identify and label the cranial cavity. Colour it purple.
- ☐ Identify and label the abdominal cavity. Colour it green.
- ☐ Identify and label the spinal cavity. Colour the spinal cord orange and the vertebrae pink.

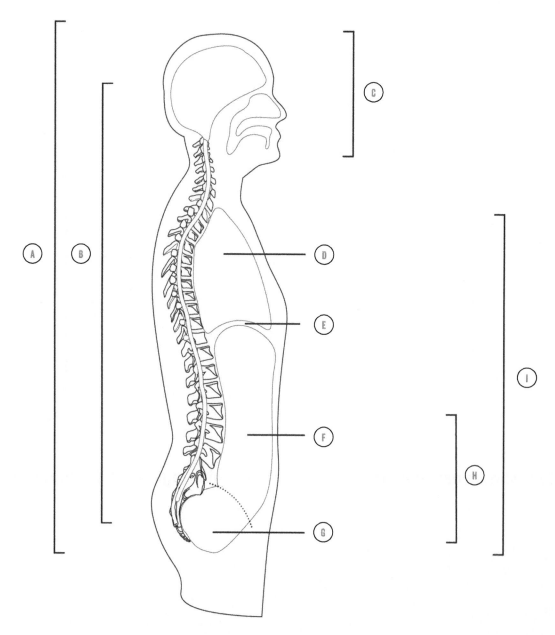

CHAPTER 2

HOMEOSTASIS IN PERSON-CENTRED PRACTICE

INTRODUCTION

The Person-Centred Practice (PCP) Framework (McCormack and McCance, 2017) is an integrated approach to people who need healthcare. It emphasises the importance of focusing on the unique characteristics of the individual in assessing need and planning and providing care. It is based on the primary concept of personhood which emphasises the importance of the individual with their own characteristics, values, beliefs and attitudes, their own life story and future plans. Person-centred practice necessitates knowledge and understanding of the individuality of the person.

Biological characteristics also vary between individuals and understanding how the human body functions is equally essential for providing high-quality care. However, the approach used within the PCP Framework tends to be seen as focusing primarily on individuals' unique psychological, social, spiritual and environmental characteristics. In providing person-centred care it is essential to integrate and coordinate all the different components of care for the person. The biological functioning of an individual influences psychological, social and spiritual responses and vice versa. This chapter will help you to revise the PCP Framework to maximise your familiarity with it. It will also help you to refresh your knowledge on homeostasis. Remember to revise Chapter 1 in *Essentials of Anatomy and Physiology for Nursing Practice*.

Answers to the labelling exercises can be found at the back of the book.

McCormack, B. and McCance, T. (2017) *Person-centred Practice in Nursing and Health Care: Theory and Practice* (2nd Edition). Chichester: Wiley-Blackwell.

THE PERSON-CENTRED PRACTICE (PCP) FRAMEWORK

INTRODUCTION

The PCP Framework is made up of layers, working from the outermost layer in. The macro context considers the strategic, political, social, educational and professional drivers that directly and indirectly impact on all other components of the PCP Framework. The prerequisites are those attributes of the nurse that are required before being able to provide high-quality person-centred care. The third layer in this model identifies a number of factors within the care environment which influence the quality of care provided and the experiences and reactions of the staff, persons being cared for and visitors. The processes in PCP are identified in the five 'petals' of the Framework. These all interact and are essential in the provision of holistic care. We are going to take the Framework apart in order to help you put it together.

——— COLOURING NOTES 2.1 ———

This diagram will deal with the first three layers of the PCP Framework. Label the three layers in the spaces provided.

Identify where the following components of the Framework belong and colour the section of the diagram to correspond:

- ☐ Appropriate skill mix - pink.
- ☐ Clarity of beliefs and values - ar green.
- ☐ Commitment to the job - light brown.
- ☐ Developed interpersonal skills - purple.
- ☐ Effective staff relationships - magenta.
- ☐ Health and social care policy - cream.
- ☐ Knowing self - red.
- ☐ Potential for innovation and risk-taking - yellow.
- ☐ Power sharing - black.
- ☐ Professionally competent - light blue.
- ☐ Shared decision making systems - grey.
- ☐ Strategic frameworks - orange.
- ☐ Strategic leadership - light green.
- ☐ Supportive organisational systems - dark brown.
- ☐ The physical environment - white.
- ☐ Workforce developments - dark blue.

See p. 5 of *Essentials of Anatomy and Physiology for Nursing Practice* to check the answers.

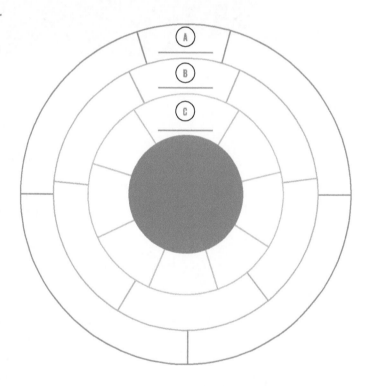

——— COLOURING NOTES 2.2 ———

This diagram will deal with the final two layers of the PCP Framework. Label the two layers in the spaces provided.

Identify where the follow components of the Framework belong and colour the section of the diagram to correspond:

- ☐ Being sympathetically present - purple.
- ☐ Engaging authentically - green.
- ☐ Existence of a healthful culture - blue.
- ☐ Feeling of well-being - yellow.
- ☐ Good care experience - orange.
- ☐ Involvement in care - red.
- ☐ Providing holistic care - magenta.
- ☐ Shared decision making - brown.
- ☐ Working with the patient's beliefs and values - pink.

See p. 5 of *Essentials of Anatomy and Physiology for Nursing Practice* to check the answers.

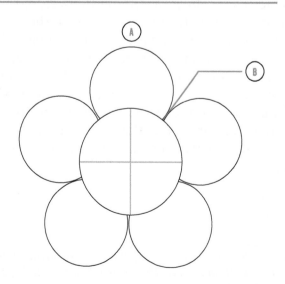

Both figures adapted from McCormack and McCance, *Person-Centred Practice in Nursing and Health Care: Theory and Practice*, 2nd Edition (2016), Wiley-Blackwell.

The Nurse's Anatomy and Physiology Colouring Book published 2017 by SAGE Publishing. © Jennifer Boore, Neal Cook and Andrea Shepherd.

BODY SYSTEMS IN HOMEOSTASIS

INTRODUCTION

The human body consists of a number of body systems which contribute to the maintenance of homeostasis through interacting to undertake necessary functions that balance out a variety of factors within the body. A good understanding of the body, its functions and organisation will enable you to provide appropriate care and to help people to maintain their own health.

COLOURING NOTES 2.3

Look at the descriptions of systems and the categories. Insert the following systems into the correct space to match the description and category:

☐ Cardiovascular system.
☐ Endocrine system.
☐ Gastrointestinal system.
☐ Immune system.
☐ Integument.
☐ Muscular system.

☐ Musculoskeletal system.
☐ Nervous system.
☐ Renal system.
☐ Reproductive system.
☐ Respiratory system.
☐ Skeletal system.

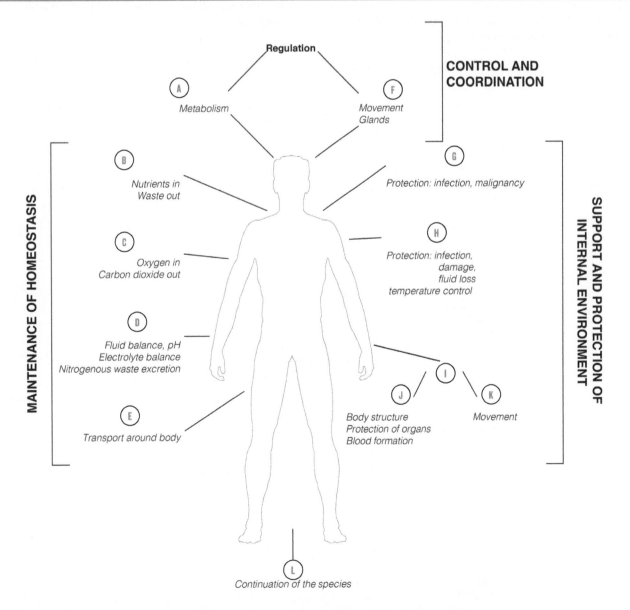

Regulation

CONTROL AND COORDINATION

A — Metabolism

F — Movement Glands

MAINTENANCE OF HOMEOSTASIS

B — Nutrients in Waste out

C — Oxygen in Carbon dioxide out

D — Fluid balance, pH Electrolyte balance Nitrogenous waste excretion

E — Transport around body

G — Protection: infection, malignancy

H — Protection: infection, damage, fluid loss temperature control

J — I — K
Body structure Protection of organs Blood formation — Movement

SUPPORT AND PROTECTION OF INTERNAL ENVIRONMENT

L — Continuation of the species

FEEDBACK SYSTEM

INTRODUCTION

The core concept in relation to physiological aspects of the individual is homeostasis and all the biological systems of the body contribute to this. So what is meant by homeostasis? In brief, homeostasis is the property of maintaining equilibrium – a stable (or nearly stable) condition of the different properties in the body (for example, body temperature, blood glucose level) through the action of the different bodily systems. In order to understand how the body functions to maintain homeostasis it is necessary to comprehend feedback and how it balances the levels of the different parameters so important for life. There are two types of feedback, positive and negative.

COLOURING NOTES 2.4

- ☐ Use one of the diagrams below to represent negative feedback. Add in the three main components of a feedback system into the boxes and add the directions of the arrows.
- ☐ Colour the effector box yellow.
- ☐ Colour the control centre box blue.
- ☐ Colour the receptor box red.
- ☐ On the dotted line beside Set Point, draw a line to illustrate variation from the set point in negative feedback.
- ☐ Use the other diagram below to represent positive feedback. Add in the three main components of a

feedback system into the boxes and add the directions of the arrows.
- ☐ Colour the effector box green.
- ☐ Colour the control centre box purple.
- ☐ Colour the receptor box orange.
- ☐ On the dotted line beside Set Point, draw a line to illustrate variation from the set point in positive feedback.

See p. 12 of Essentials of Anatomy and Physiology for Nursing Practice to check the answers

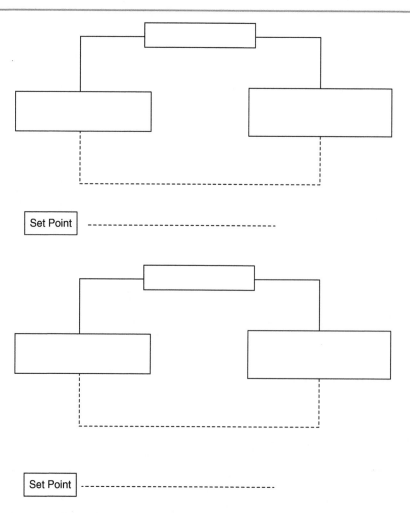

CHAPTER 3

THE HUMAN CELL

INTRODUCTION

During the life of every individual, the balance in the cells of which they are composed goes through various stages. Cell multiplication increases the number of body cells while apoptosis (programmed cell death) reduces this number. Both processes occur throughout life but the balance between them varies and permits normal growth and development. The two types of cell division are:

- **mitosis** for growth and repair of tissues,
- **meiosis** for creation of sperm or ova (gametes) containing half the normal genetic material for formation of the next generation.

Cells initially have the potential to differentiate into any type of body cell – they are known as stem cells and, while most become fixed as a particular type of cell, some retain their flexibility and continue in certain tissues as stem cells. Cells with the ability to develop into any of the cells which make up the body are known as pluripotent stem cells (e.g. embryonic stem cells); those which are more limited but able to form more than one cell type are known as multipotent (e.g. adult stem cells and cord blood cells). In this chapter, you will review the structure of the cell and its components and you will also revise cellular division. Remember to review Chapter 2 in *Essentials of Anatomy and Physiology for Nursing Practice*.

Answers to the labelling exercises can be found at the back of the book.

ANATOMY OF A HUMAN CELL

INTRODUCTION

The human (mammalian) cell is a complex structure able to carry out all the functions required to maintain cell life and also makes its contribution to homeostasis through the activities of the different organelles (small organs) within the cell.

COLOURING NOTES 3.1

- ☐ Identify and label the following:
  - ○ Ribosomes
  - ○ Centrioles
  - ○ Nucleus
  - ○ Golgi apparatus
  - ○ Smooth endoplasmic reticulum
  - ○ Rough endoplasmic reticulum
  - ○ Mitochondrion
  - ○ Centrosomes
  - ○ Cell membrane
  - ○ Nuclear membrane
  - ○ Secretory granules
  - ○ Nucleolus.
- ☐ Colour the nucleolus black.
- ☐ Colour the cytoplasm of the nucleus yellow.
- ☐ Colour the cytoplasm of the cell blue.
- ☐ Colour the secretory granules orange.
- ☐ Colour the Golgi apparatus pink.
- ☐ Colour the mitochondria green.
- ☐ Colour the smooth endoplasmic reticulum red.
- ☐ Colour the rough endoplasmic reticulum brown.

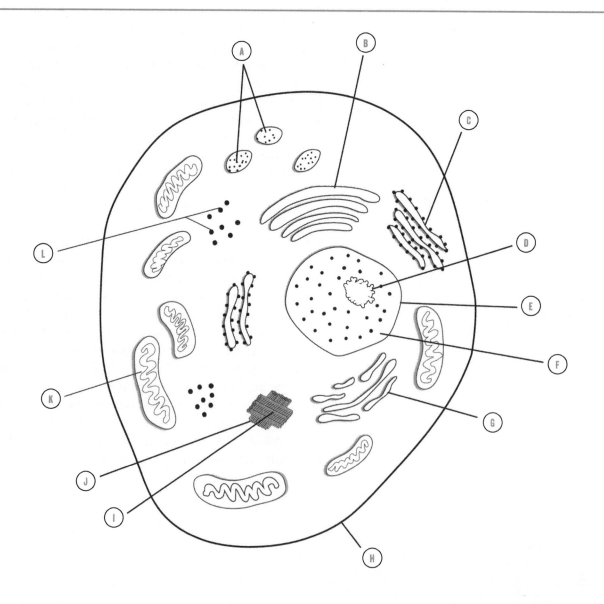

DNA STRUCTURE

INTRODUCTION

Chromosomes are formed of two DNA strands with backbones of alternating sugar (deoxyribose) and phosphate molecules connected by pairs of nitrogen-containing bases, two purine (adenine and guanine) and two pyrimidine (thymine and cytosine); a purine always connects with a pyrimidine. Adenine joins with thymine by two chemical bonds, and guanine connects with cytosine by three chemical bonds.

——— COLOURING NOTES 3.2 ———

Think about how the bases pair up and the number of chemical bonds between them. In the diagram below, use the letter A to represent Adenine, G to represent Guanine, T to represent Thymine and C to represent Cytosine. Match these pairs of bases up correctly by inserting the correct letter in the correct space between the hydrogen bonds.

- ☐ Colour the adenine bases purple.
- ☐ Colour the thymine bases red.
- ☐ Colour the cytosine bases yellow.
- ☐ Colour the guanine bases green.
- ☐ In the diagram you will see that CH_2 bonds with another unlabelled substance. Identify that substance and label it with the first letter of its name. Colour these blue.

See p. 22 of *Essentials of Anatomy and Physiology for Nursing Practice* to check the answers.

- ☐ Choose a colour for cytosine and colour all the cytosine segments. Colour the empty circle beside the label for cytosine so that your colour choice is clear.
- ☐ Which of the three other substances identified below the image pairs with cytosine? Choose a colour for it and colour the correct segments. Colour the empty circle beside the label for that substance so that your colour choice is clear.
- ☐ Choose a colour for adenine and colour all the adenine segments. Colour the empty circle beside the label for adenine so that your colour choice is clear.
- ☐ There will be one of the four substances identified below the image not paired up. Choose a colour for it and colour the correct segments. Colour the empty circle beside the label for that substance so that your colour choice is clear.

See p. 22 of *Essentials of Anatomy and Physiology for Nursing Practice* to check the answers.

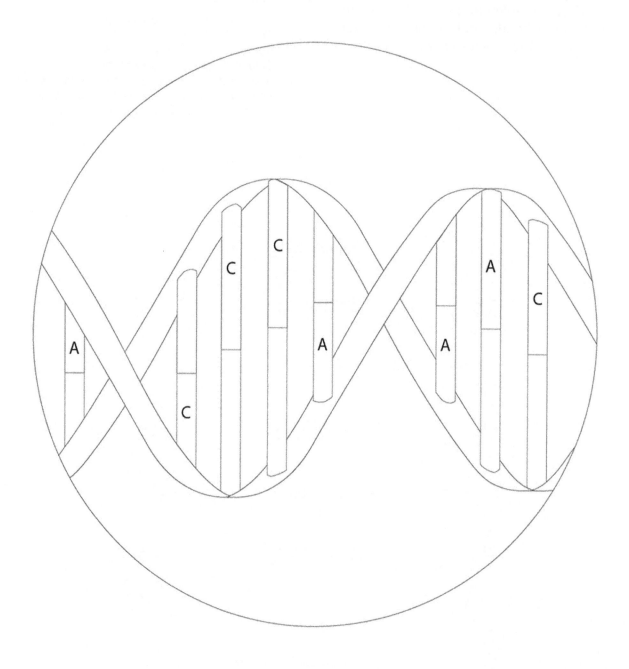

○ Cytosine   ○ Thymine   ○ Adenine   ○ Guanine

PROTEIN FORMATION

INTRODUCTION

DNA in the chromosomes carries the genetic material that determines the individual's characteristics. It does this by acting as a template for the formation of the proteins of the body from the amino acids (the nutrients absorbed into the body after the breakdown of proteins in the diet). This determines both structure and function of the components of the body. The process occurs in two main stages:

1. Transcription of DNA to Ribonucleic Acid (RNA).
2. Translation (to proteins).

COLOURING NOTES 3.3

☐ Identify and label the following:
  ○ Ribosome
  ○ Nuclear membrane
  ○ Nuclear pore
  ○ Nucleus
  ○ Amino acids forming a protein chain

  ○ DNA
  ○ mRNA.
☐ Colour the cytoplasm of the nucleus yellow.
☐ Colour the cytoplasm of the cell blue.
☐ Colour the ribosome brown.
☐ Colour the amino acids red.

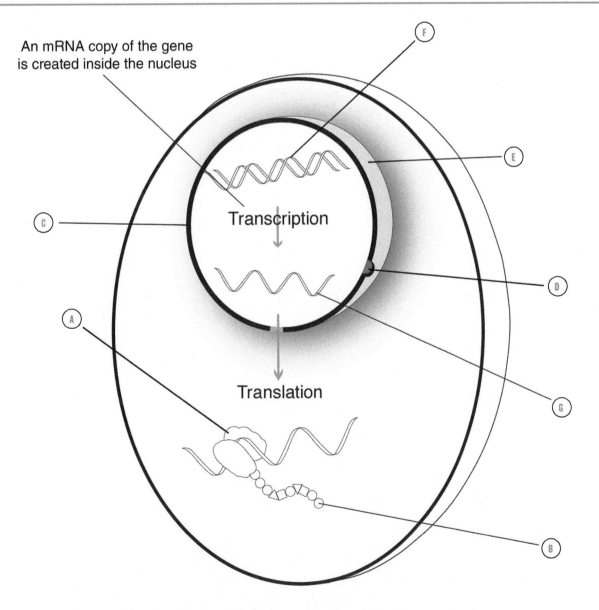

An mRNA copy of the gene is created inside the nucleus

Transcription

Translation

CELL MEMBRANE

INTRODUCTION

The boundary of each cell is a double-layered lipid membrane, the cell or plasma membrane, composed of phospholipids (fatty molecules with a phosphate group), proteins and carbohydrates arranged in a mosaic structure. The phosphate ends of phospholipids are attracted to water (hydrophilic) and they face outwards from the cell membrane while the fatty acid tails are water repellent (hydrophobic) and face each other in the centre of the membrane, preventing passage of all but very small molecules.

COLOURING NOTES 3.4

☐ Identify and label the following:
  ○ Carbohydrate chain
  ○ Intrinsic membrane proteins.
☐ Colour the intrinsic membrane proteins green.

☐ Colour the carbohydrate chain yellow.
☐ Colour the phosphate ends of the phospholipids purple.
☐ Colour the fatty acid tails of the phospholipids red.

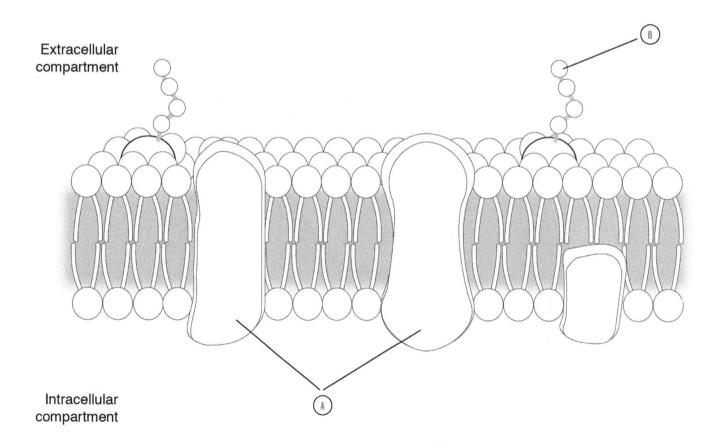

Extracellular compartment

Intracellular compartment

TRANSPORT ACROSS THE CELL MEMBRANE

INTRODUCTION

The cell membrane controls how substances can move in and out of the cell. Carrier proteins facilitate the movement of specific molecules. These are proteins which pass through the cell membrane and provide a site recognised by specific molecules which link to it. The protein then changes conformation and releases the molecule on the other side of the membrane. The proteins assist movement of substances by what is known as carrier-mediated transport, requiring energy.

COLOURING NOTES 3.5

☐ Identify and label the following:
  ○ Carrier proteins
  ○ Substances to be transported.

☐ Colour the carrier proteins green.
☐ Colour the substances to be transported yellow.
☐ Colour the phospholipids blue.

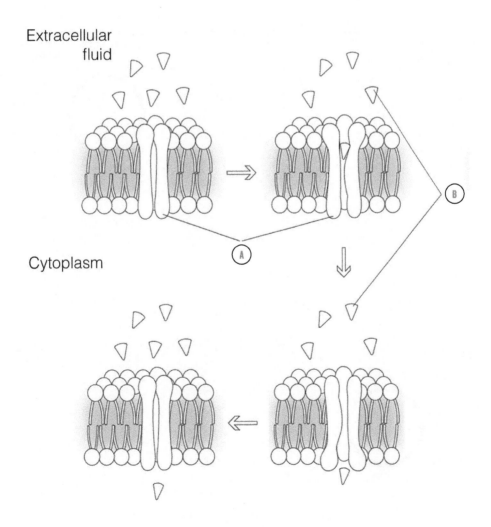

Extracellular fluid

Cytoplasm

A

B

ENDOCYTOSIS AND EXOCYTOSIS

INTRODUCTION

Exocytosis and endocytosis enable large molecules that cannot pass though the cell membrane to move between the intracellular fluid and extracellular fluid. Endocytosis enables molecules to enter the cell by engulfing it. Exocytosis enables the contents of a vesicle formed from the Golgi apparatus to fuse with the cell membrane and the contents are released from the cell.

COLOURING NOTES 3.6

- ☐ Identify which of the two images below is exocytosis and which is endocytosis and label them.
- ☐ Identify the substances entering and leaving the cell and colour them orange.
- ☐ Draws arrows to show the correct direction of movement between the different stages in each image.
- ☐ Colour the cytoplasm blue.
- ☐ Identify and label the vesicles and colour their margins yellow.

See p. 29 of *Essentials of Anatomy and Physiology for Nursing Practice* to check the answers.

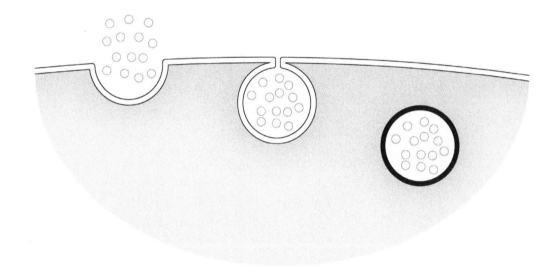

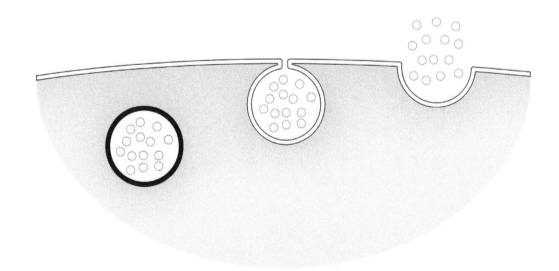

MEIOSIS AND MITOSIS

INTRODUCTION

Meiosis occurs in relation to reproduction and is the division that occurs to form the gametes – sperm or ova – in preparation for fertilisation and formation of the zygote which develops into the foetus. The gamete from each parent normally contains half the full number of chromosomes (i.e. 23:22 autosomes and one sex chromosome).

——— COLOURING NOTES 3.7 ———

☐ Identify and label the chromosomes. Colour these orange.
☐ Identify and label where the sister chromatids separate. Colour these red.
☐ Identify and label the gametes. Colour these blue.
☐ Identify and label the sister chromatids. Colour these yellow.
☐ Identify where the homologues separate (sisters remain attached) and colour these green.

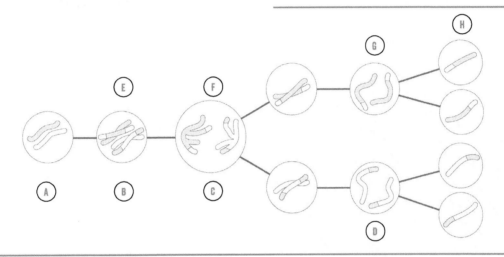

Mitosis is when a cell divides into two genetically identical daughter cells. Continued cell division occurs as the body develops through various stages. It also enables tissue repair.

Mitosis consists of five main stages (but not in this order):

- Telophase.
- Metaphase.
- Anaphase.
- Interphase.
- Prophase.

——— COLOURING NOTES 3.8 ———

☐ Label the five phases of mitosis correctly on the diagram.
☐ Colour the chromatids in the prophase and metaphase stages red.
☐ Identify in which step the chromatids separate and colour them yellow.
☐ Colour the chromosomes in the telophase stage green.
☐ Colour the homologous chromosomes in the interphase stage orange.

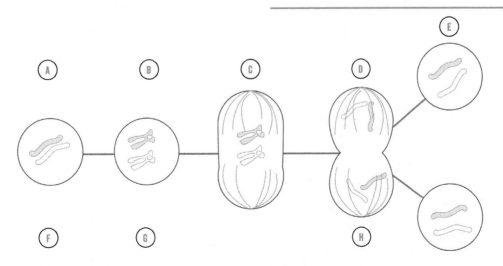

CARTILAGE

INTRODUCTION

Cartilage is firmer than other connective tissues with fewer cells (chondrocytes) within a substantial matrix. There are three types of cartilage:

- Hyaline.
- Fibrocartilage.
- Elastic fibrocartilage.

—— COLOURING NOTES 3.9 ——

- ☐ Identify which type of cartilage is represented in each image and label them correctly.
- ☐ Label the chondrocytes in each image and colour them blue.
- ☐ Identify and label the solid matrix. Colour it yellow.
- ☐ Identify and label the collagen fibres. Colour them orange.
- ☐ Identify and label the elastic fibres. Colour them pink.
- ☐ Identify and label a cell nest.

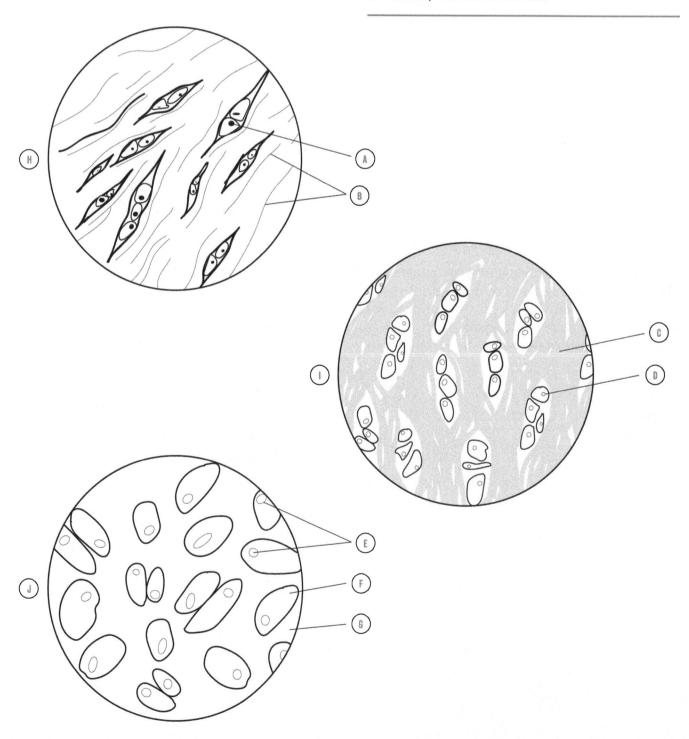

CHAPTER 4

THE HUMAN MICROBIOME AND HEALTH

INTRODUCTION

More than 90% of the cells in the human body are not human in origin but microbial, that is, only visible under a microscope. They form the microbiome and are an integral part of the human body. In this chapter you will review the major groups of microbes within and on the human body and their structure. Remember to revise Chapter 4 in *Essentials of Anatomy and Physiology for Nursing Practice*.

Answers to the labelling exercises can be found at the back of the book.

BACTERIA

INTRODUCTION

Bacteria are the most important microbes in the context of the human microbiome. They are single-celled prokaryotes; the major difference from eukaryotes is that the cell organelles in bacteria are not enclosed by cell membrane but lie directly within the cytoplasm: they do not have an enclosed nucleus.

COLOURING NOTES 4.1

☐ Identify and label the following:
- ○ Flagellum
- ○ Ribosomes
- ○ DNA
- ○ Cytoplasm
- ○ Pilus
- ○ Cytoplasmic membrane
- ○ Cell wall.

☐ Colour the cytoplasmic membrane green.
☐ Colour the cytoplasm yellow.
☐ Colour the cell wall blue.

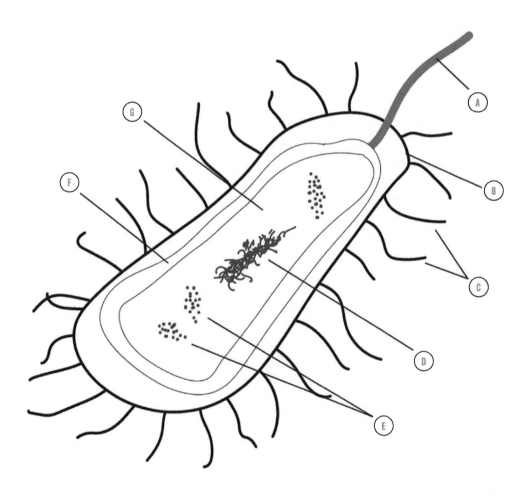

SHAPES OF BACTERIA

INTRODUCTION

The following are used to describe the shape and organisation of bacteria:

- Round (coccus) which exist individually and in pairs, chains and clusters.
- Rod (bacillus) which also exist individually and in chains.
- Curved (vibrio) individuals.
- Spiral (spirochaete) individuals.

COLOURING NOTES 4.2

- ☐ Identify, label and colour the spirochaetes orange.
- ☐ Identify and label a single coccus. Colour it green.
- ☐ Identify, label and colour the vibrios brown.
- ☐ Identify and label the coccobacilli. Colour them pink.
- ☐ Identify and label the diplococci. Colour them red.
- ☐ Identify and label the streptococci. Colour them yellow.
- ☐ Identify and label a single bacillus. Colour it purple.
- ☐ Identify and label the staphylococci. Colour them blue.

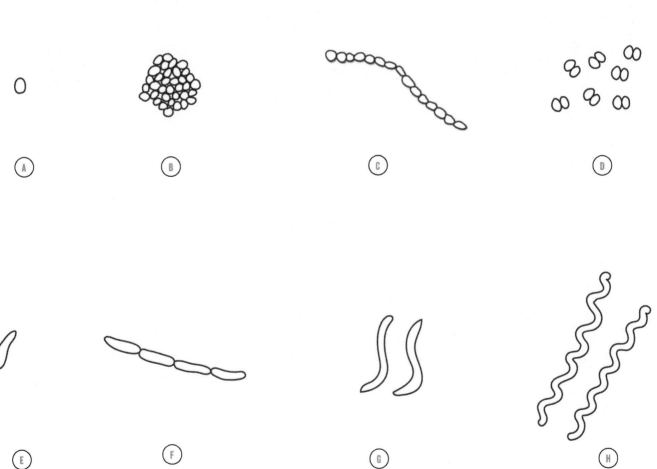

SPECIALISED STRUCTURES OF BACTERIA

INTRODUCTION

The following characteristics are used to describe the structure of bacteria by the presence or absence of specialised structures:

- Mucous capsule protects against dehydration and desiccation in dry conditions.
- Flagella enable bacteria to move.
- Spore formation occurs in some bacteria under adverse conditions with germination and cell division recommencing when conditions improve.
- Pili provide attachment to the host.

COLOURING NOTES 4.3

- ☐ Identify and label the flagellated bacteria. Colour them green.
- ☐ Colour the fimbriated bacterium pink.
- ☐ Identify and label the encapsulated diplococci. Colour them blue and the mucus yellow.
- ☐ Identify and label the encapsulated bacilli. Colour them brown and the mucus green.
- ☐ Identify and label the bacillus with spores. Label the chain and spores. Colour all the spores purple and the bacilli red.

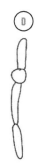

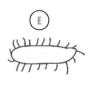

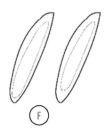

The Nurse's Anatomy and Physiology Colouring Book published 2017 by SAGE Publishing. © Jennifer Boore, Neal Cook and Andrea Shepherd.

ORGANISM GROWTH: BINARY FISSION

INTRODUCTION

The conditions for growth of bacteria vary with individual species but must meet their needs in relation to:

- Temperature.
- Moisture.
- pH level.
- Oxygen.

Different organisms will grow at different speeds and demonstrate exponential growth through binary fission as the DNA replicates and separates, and the cell divides into two identical daughter cells. The time taken for this process to occur is known as the generation time and varies with different species. Binary fission continues with the cell numbers doubling on each occasion, until the limits of the supplies of requirements for cell division are reached.

——— COLOURING NOTES 4.4 ———

- ☐ Identify and label a chromosome.
- ☐ Identify the daughter cells and colour them green.
- ☐ Identify the mother cell and colour it red.
- ☐ Identify the stage where the DNA molecules separate and colour the cell blue.
- ☐ Identify the stage where the cell lengthens and duplicates its DNA. Colour it purple.
- ☐ Identify the stage of cross wall formation and colour the cell/cells orange.

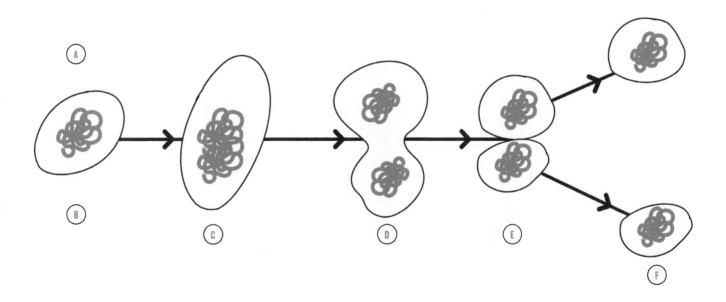

EXAMPLES OF VIRUSES

INTRODUCTION

Viruses are intracellular parasites without independent life outside the cells they infect; all life is host to one or more viruses. Viruses vary in shape and size and, in their simplest form, consist of the genetic material of nucleic acid (either DNA or RNA) surrounded by a protein capsule. Some are further surrounded by a membrane envelope.

—————————————————— COLOURING NOTES 4.5 ——————————————————

☐ Identify and label the following in the bacteriophage:
  ○ Fibres
  ○ Nucleic acid
  ○ Protein coat
  ○ Tail (sheath)
  ○ DNA.

☐ Colour the nucleic acid yellow.
☐ Colour the protein coat blue.
☐ Colour the fibres green.
☐ Colour the tail (sheath) purple.
☐ Trace along the DNA in black.

Bacteriophage
(DNA Virus)

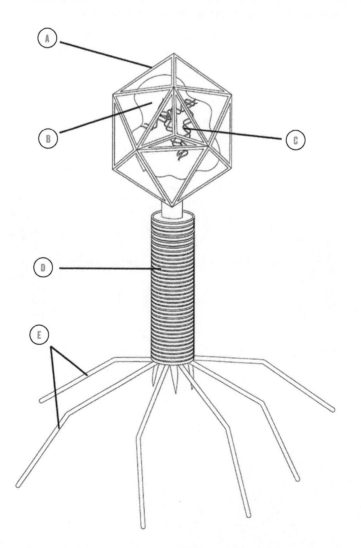

COLOURING NOTES 4.6

☐ Identify and label the following in the influenza virus:

    ○ Protein coat
    ○ Membrane envelope
    ○ RNA.

☐ Colour the protein coat green.
☐ Colour the membrane envelope yellow.
☐ Trace along the RNA in black.
☐ Colour the remaining elements in colours of your choice.

Influenza

(RNA Virus)

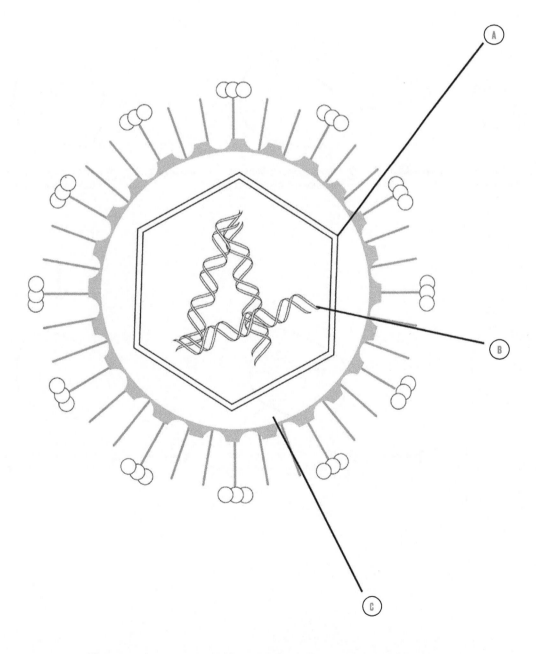

LIFE CYCLE OF A VIRUS

INTRODUCTION

Viruses multiply within the cells of their host and are then released into their environment. There are six stages to this process.

--- COLOURING NOTES 4.7 ---

☐ Identify the virus capsules present across all of the stages. Colour it orange everywhere you can locate it.
☐ Identify and label the following (of the host cell):
  ○ Cell membrane
  ○ Cytoplasm
  ○ Cell nucleus containing DNA.
☐ Colour the cytoplasm of the cell green.
☐ Colour the nucleus of the cell yellow.

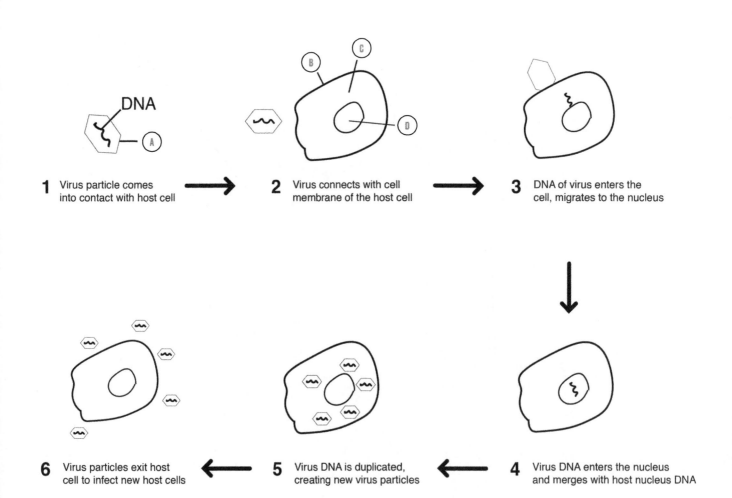

1 Virus particle comes into contact with host cell

2 Virus connects with cell membrane of the host cell

3 DNA of virus enters the cell, migrates to the nucleus

6 Virus particles exit host cell to infect new host cells

5 Virus DNA is duplicated, creating new virus particles

4 Virus DNA enters the nucleus and merges with host nucleus DNA

FUNGI

INTRODUCTION

These are eukaryotes but are neither plants nor animals. Some have a simple structure and exist as unicellular organisms, for example yeasts. Others are more complex and exist as a mycelium, an interwoven mat of tubular filaments or hyphae. Some fungi are found in healthy individuals but can cause disease if the environment becomes compromised.

COLOURING NOTES 4.8

- ☐ Identify and label at least one nucleus in each of the images. Colour all the nuclei yellow.
- ☐ Identify and label the spore and its tough wall. Colour it pink.
- ☐ Colour the budding yeasts blue.
- ☐ Colour the cytoplasm of the mycelium green.
- ☐ Identify and label the hyphae.

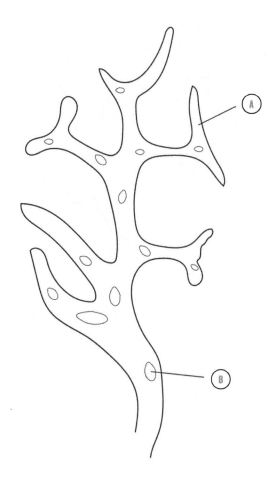

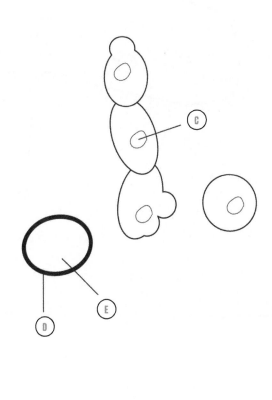

PROTOZOA

INTRODUCTION

Protozoa/protists are unicellular microorganisms most of which are harmless, but some are pathogens or opportunists. Examples of particularly unpleasant GIT pathogens are *Cryptosporidium* and *Giardia*.

COLOURING NOTES 4.9

- ☐ Identify and label which image is the:
  - ○ Amoeba
  - ○ Paramecium
  - ○ Euglena.
- ☐ Identify and label the following:
  - ○ Flagellum
  - ○ Cilia
  - ○ Pseudopod.

- ☐ Colour the cytoplasm of the cells blue.
- ☐ Colour the contractile vacuoles (star shaped structures) yellow.
- ☐ Colour the nuclei orange.
- ☐ Colour the remaining structures in colours of your choice.

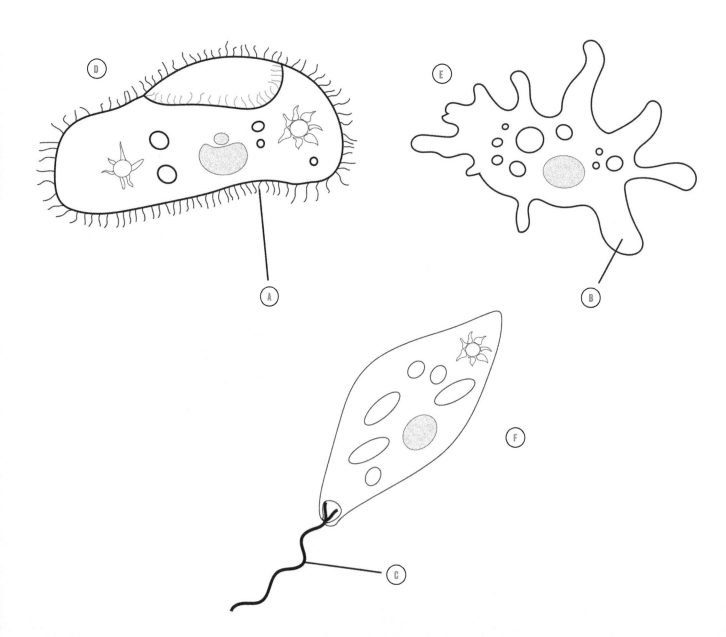

HELMINTHS (WORMS)

INTRODUCTION

Helminths (worms) are uncommon residents of the human gut in developed countries but more common where contamination of water and food is prevalent. While the idea of having worms resident in one's gut is unpleasant, some may have certain health benefits particularly in relation to allergic disorders.

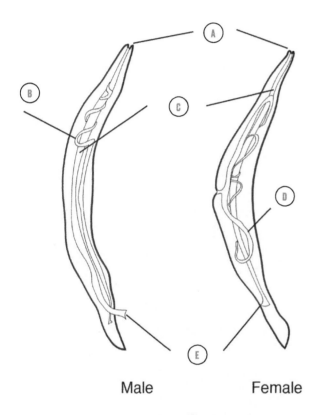

Male   Female

Round worm

—— COLOURING NOTES 4.10 ——

- ☐ Identify and label the mouth and anus in both images.
- ☐ Identify and label the intestine in both images. Colour it orange in both.
- ☐ Identify and label the ovary in the female. Colour it pink.
- ☐ Identify and label the testis in the male. Colour it yellow.
- ☐ Colour the remainder of the round worm blue.

—— COLOURING NOTES 4.11 ——

- ☐ Identify label the hooks and a sucker. Colour the suckers orange
- ☐ Identify and label the tapes. Colour them yellow.
- ☐ Identify and label the head. Colour it pink.
- ☐ Identify and label the neck. Colour it blue.
- ☐ Colour the image of the whole worm (to the right) brown.

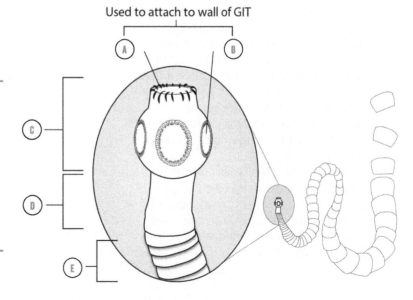

Used to attach to wall of GIT

MICROBIOME, HEALTH AND DISEASE

INTRODUCTION

In recent years, researchers have identified relationships between the human microbiome and a variety of human diseases. Not unexpectedly, some relationships between the microbiome and some intestinal disorders, for example, Inflammatory Bowel Disease (IBD) have been identified. However, a number of other disorders have also been linked to the gut microbes.

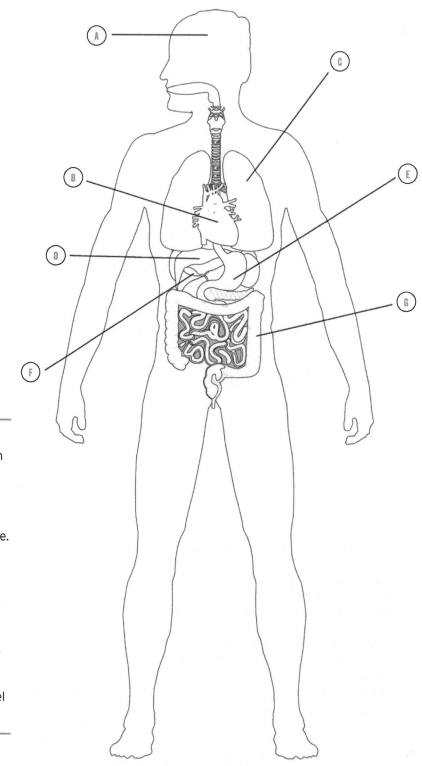

— COLOURING NOTES 4.12 —

- ☐ Identify and label the organ involved with bile circulation. Colour it green.
- ☐ Identify and label the organ linked with cardiovascular disorders. Colour it red.
- ☐ Identify and label the organ linked with allergic breathing disorders. Colour it blue.
- ☐ Identify and label the organ linked with drug metabolism. Colour it purple.
- ☐ Identify and label the organ linked with mood/mental health disorders. Colour its location yellow.
- ☐ Identify and label the organ linked with malnutrition and obesity. Colour it green.
- ☐ Identify and label the organ associated with being in contact with carcinogenic food substances and inflammatory bowel disease. Colour it pink.

SKIN

INTRODUCTION

The skin is the body's largest organ (approximately 1.8–2 m²) and is the interface with the external environment. The skin has its own ecosystem with a wide range of resident microbes including bacteria, viruses, fungi and, sometimes, mites. The rough texture of the epidermis means that many microbes can be resident in the different grooves of papillae, in hair follicles and in ducts of sweat glands. Most of these are commensals and protect against invasion by non-resident flora through action on sweat, partly by producing fatty acids which inhibit growth of fungi. Mites reside in the areas where hair covers the skin and are considered part of the normal flora, although they can sometimes cause skin disorders. The average adult has approximately 1,000 species of bacteria colonised on their skin, amounting to about 1 trillion bacteria, but the good news is that, largely, we are immune to our own skin microflora

─── **COLOURING NOTES 4.13** ───

- ☐ Identify and label the two blank sections to the left of the diagram.
- ☐ Identify the hairs in the skin. Colour them brown.
- ☐ Identify the sweat pores and glands. Colour them pink.
- ☐ Identify the adipose tissue. Colour it yellow.

- ☐ Shade the dermis in blue.
- ☐ Shade the epidermis in green.
- ☐ Identify and colour the arteries red.
- ☐ Identify and colour the veins purple.

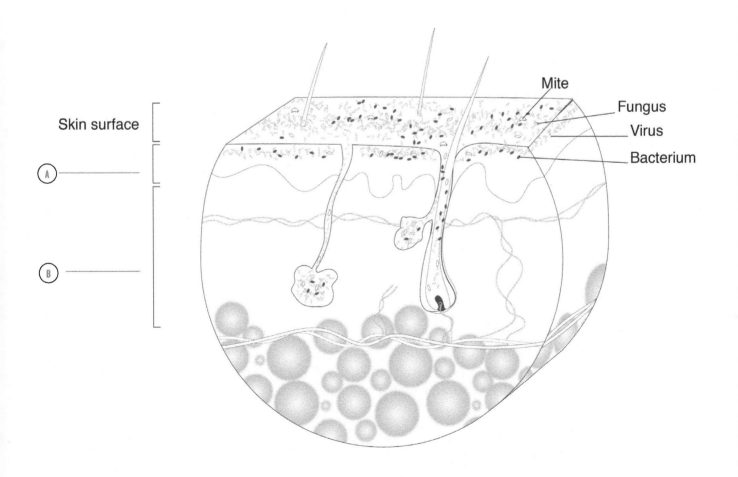

CHAPTER 5

THE NERVOUS SYSTEM: CONTROL OF BODY FUNCTION

INTRODUCTION

The nervous system is central to who we are as functioning, living, feeling people. It shapes who we are, how we experience life and how we function physically, socially and emotionally. As we go through the journey of life, the nervous system develops, and continues to develop, coordinating our development, influencing our life choices and cataloguing our experiences. This chapter will help you to revise the structure and function of the nervous system. You will have learned about cells of the nervous system (neurons and neuroglia), how they communicate through transmission of nervous impulses and support each other, and how the nervous system is structurally and biochemically protected. You will also return to the structural and functional divisions of the nervous system. Remember to revise Chapter 5 in *Essentials of Anatomy and Physiology for Nursing Practice*.

Answers to the labelling exercises can be found at the back of the book.

STRUCTURE OF A NEURON

INTRODUCTION

Neurons are how electrical messages are sent around the body. They are often referred to as nerve cells, being one of the two mains types of cells in the nervous system. There are three types of neurons: motor, sensory and interneurons. Below is a motor neuron which carries electrical messages from the central nervous system to an effector (e.g. muscle).

COLOURING NOTES 5.1

☐   Identify and label the nucleus. Colour it black.
☐   Identify and label the dendrites, axon terminal, and nodes of Ranvier.
☐   Identify and label the neurofibrils. Colour them yellow.
☐   Label the axon and colour the cytoplasm of the cell (liquid inside the cell) blue.
☐   Colour the Schwann cells red.

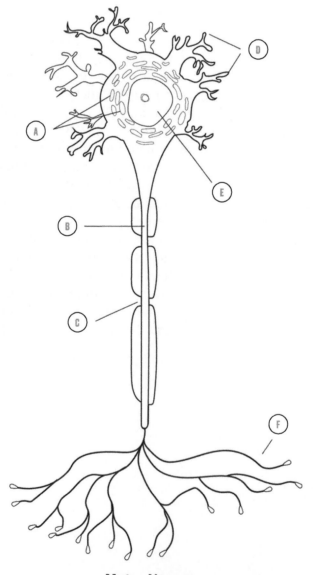

Motor Neuron

SYNAPTIC TRANSMISSION

INTRODUCTION

Synaptic transmission is how action potentials (nervous impulses) are communicated from one neuron to another. This can be electrical or chemical.

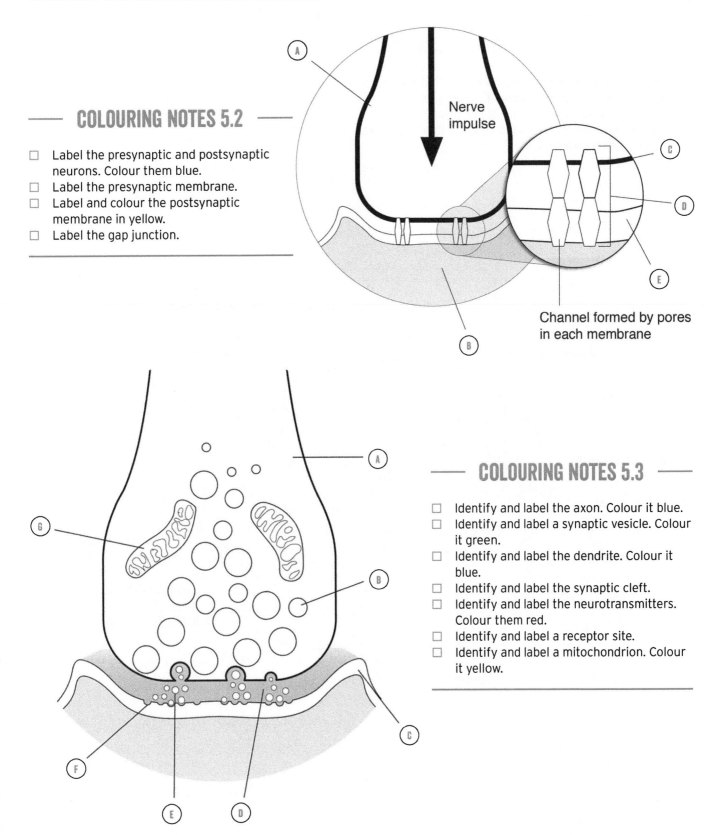

— COLOURING NOTES 5.2 —

☐ Label the presynaptic and postsynaptic neurons. Colour them blue.
☐ Label the presynaptic membrane.
☐ Label and colour the postsynaptic membrane in yellow.
☐ Label the gap junction.

Nerve impulse

Channel formed by pores in each membrane

— COLOURING NOTES 5.3 —

☐ Identify and label the axon. Colour it blue.
☐ Identify and label a synaptic vesicle. Colour it green.
☐ Identify and label the dendrite. Colour it blue.
☐ Identify and label the synaptic cleft.
☐ Identify and label the neurotransmitters. Colour them red.
☐ Identify and label a receptor site.
☐ Identify and label a mitochondrion. Colour it yellow.

STRUCTURE OF THE BRAIN

INTRODUCTION

The brain is divided into three main structures; the forebrain, the midbrain and the hindbrain. Each of these structures work together to maintain homeostasis. Different parts of the brain have different roles.

--- **COLOURING NOTES 5.4** ---

☐ Identify and label the thalamus and hypothalamus. Colour the thalamus orange.
☐ Identify and label the cerebellum. Colour it purple.
☐ Identify and label the pituitary gland. Colour it yellow.
☐ Identify and label the pons and medulla oblongata. Colour these blue.
☐ Colour the forebrain green.

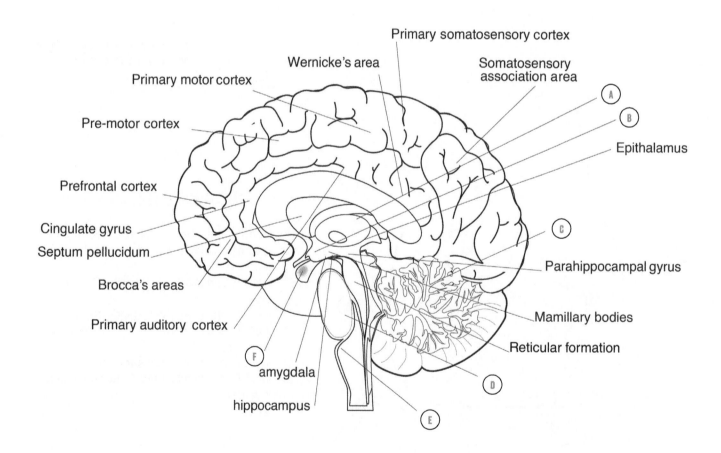

LOBES OF THE BRAIN

INTRODUCTION

The cerebrum consists of the cerebral cortex, underlying white matter, the basal nuclei and the limbic system. A deep fissure divides the cerebrum into two halves (the cerebral hemispheres). It is further divided by folds into five functional lobes.

COLOURING NOTES 5.5

☐ Identify and label the frontal lobe. Colour it red.
☐ Identify and label the occipital lobe. Colour it green.
☐ Identify and label the temporal lobe. Colour it orange.
☐ Identify and label the parietal lobe. Colour it purple.

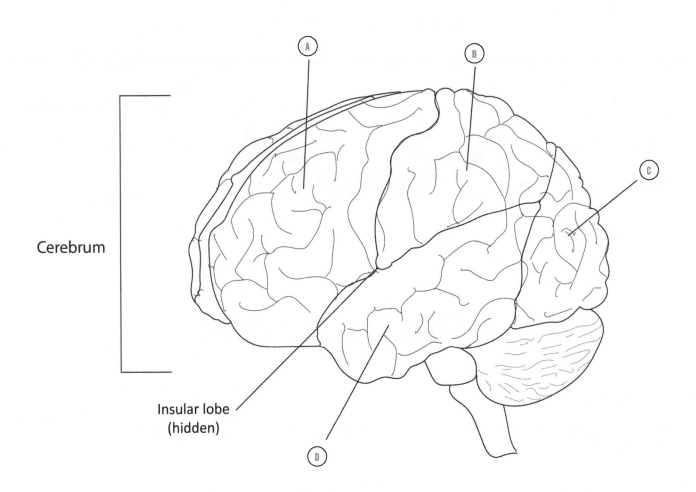

THE SPINAL CORD

INTRODUCTION

The spinal cord is the neural tissue encased within the spine which runs from the medulla, where it joins the brain at the foramen magnum, to the level of the first or second lumbar vertebrae. There are three groups of neurons which run through the spinal cord; ascending (afferent), descending (efferent) and interneurons (association neurons).

COLOURING NOTES 5.6

- ☐ Identify and label the white matter. Colour it yellow.
- ☐ Identify and label the grey matter. Colour it purple.
- ☐ Identify and label the interneuron.
- ☐ Colour in the two root ganglions in red.

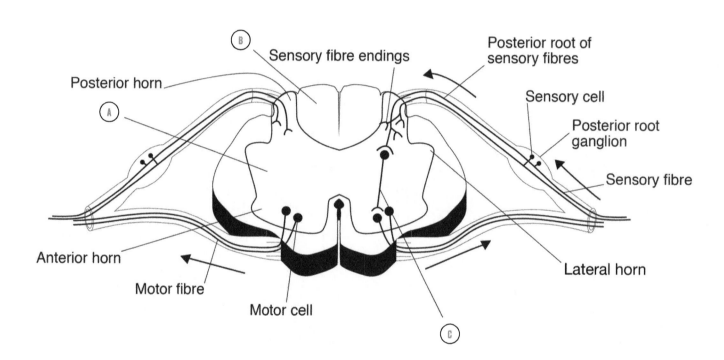

SENSORY ORDER NEURONS

INTRODUCTION

Sensory information is normally carried to the brain through three sets of neurons: first, second and third order neurons.

COLOURING NOTES 5.7

- ☐ Identify and label the first order neuron (afferent). Colour it yellow.
- ☐ Identify and label the second order neuron. Colour it orange.
- ☐ Identify and label the third order neuron. Colour it red.

Stimulus

Receptors ——

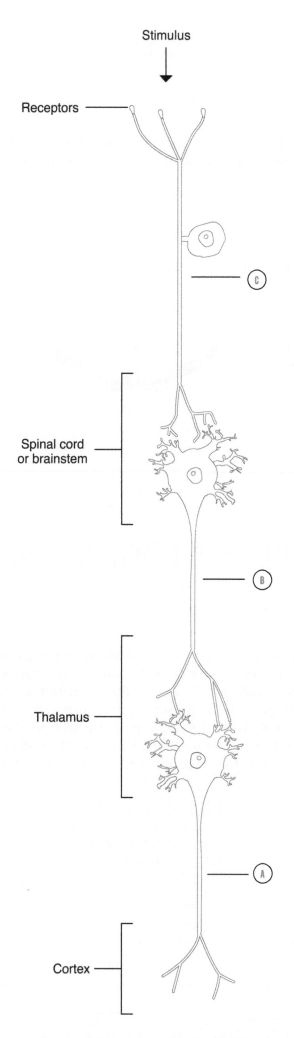

Ⓒ

Spinal cord
or brainstem ——

Ⓑ

Thalamus ——

Ⓐ

Cortex ——

The Nurse's Anatomy and Physiology Colouring Book published 2017 by SAGE Publishing. © Jennifer Boore, Neal Cook and Andrea Shepherd.

REFLEX ARC

INTRODUCTION

A reflex arc enables a very rapid response to harmful stimuli. For example, if you touch a hot iron, the simple reflex will withdraw your hand very rapidly. This is managed at the level of the spinal cord.

─── COLOURING NOTES 5.8 ───

☐ Draw arrows on the diagram indicating the direction of nervous impulse for a reflex arc.
☐ Identify and label the sensory, motor and interneurons.
☐ Colour the effector muscle orange.
☐ Colour the white matter yellow.
☐ Colour the grey matter purple.

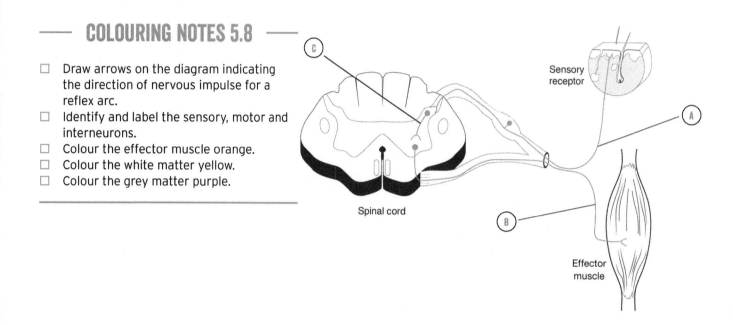

AUTONOMIC NERVOUS SYSTEM

INTRODUCTION

The autonomic nervous system is a subconscious control system for visceral organs including those of the circulatory, digestive and respiratory systems. Most of the pathways in the autonomic nervous system are motor pathways, but include some sensory pathways, indicating that the autonomic nervous system works in synergy with the sensory system in places. The autonomic nervous system has two divisions, the sympathetic and the parasympathetic nervous systems. Although anatomically and functionally different, both divisions normally stimulate the same organs. The sympathetic and parasympathetic nervous systems work in harmony to maintain homeostasis.

────── COLOURING NOTES 5.9 ──────

☐ Label the cervical, thoracic, lumbar, sacral and coccygeal nerve segments, and colour them red, green, orange, blue and yellow respectively.
☐ Draw a line from the following organs to the correct areas on

the parasympathetic division of the nervous system:
○ Lung
○ Heart
○ Liver
○ Stomach
○ Spleen

○ Pancreas
○ Small intestine
○ Large intestine
○ Bladder
○ Reproductive organs.

See p. 129 of *Essentials of Anatomy and Physiology for Nursing Practice* to check the answers.

The Nurse's Anatomy and Physiology Colouring Book published 2017 by SAGE Publishing. © Jennifer Boore, Neal Cook and Andrea Shepherd.

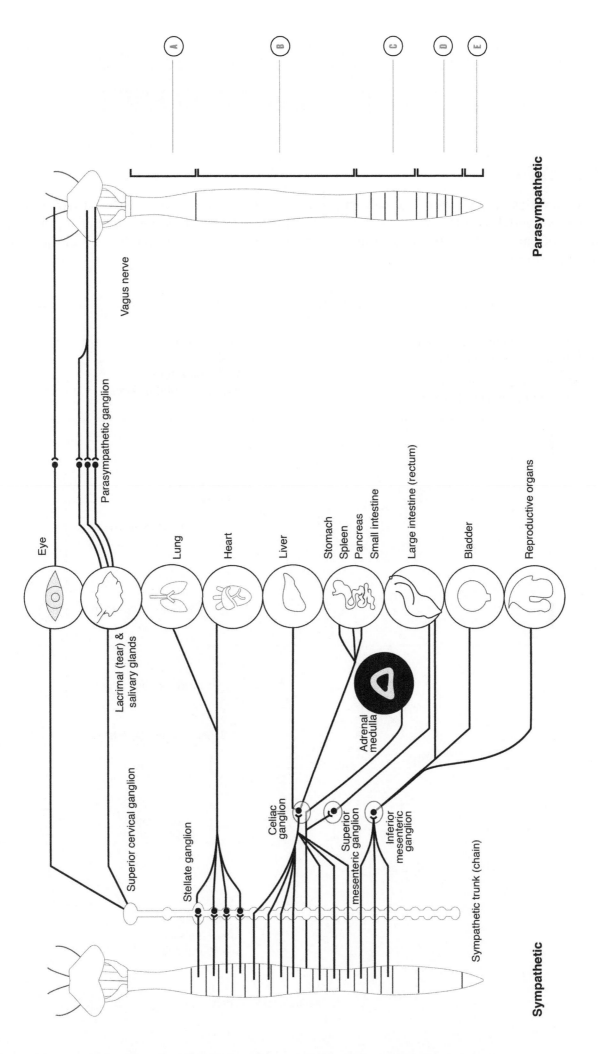

Parasympathetic

A
B
C
D
E

Vagus nerve

Parasympathetic ganglion

Eye

Lacrimal (tear) & salivary glands

Lung

Heart

Liver

Stomach
Spleen
Pancreas
Small intestine

Large intestine (rectum)

Bladder

Reproductive organs

Superior cervical ganglion

Stellate ganglion

Celiac ganglion

Superior mesenteric ganglion

Inferior mesenteric ganglion

Adrenal medulla

Sympathetic trunk (chain)

Sympathetic

NUTRITION AND PROTECTION OF THE NERVOUS SYSTEM: CEREBRAL CIRCULATION

INTRODUCTION

The main arteries supplying the brain are the two internal carotid arteries and the basilar artery (arising from the two vertebral arteries). The Circle of Willis is a circle of blood vessels that supplies blood to the different parts of the brain. It is formed from the main arteries supplying the brain joined by the connecting arteries.

--- COLOURING NOTES 5.10 ---

☐ Colour the circulatory vessels red.
☐ Identify and label the following:

  ○ Middle cerebral artery
  ○ Anterior communicating artery

  ○ Circle of Willis
  ○ Basilar artery
  ○ Vertebral artery
  ○ Internal carotid arteries.

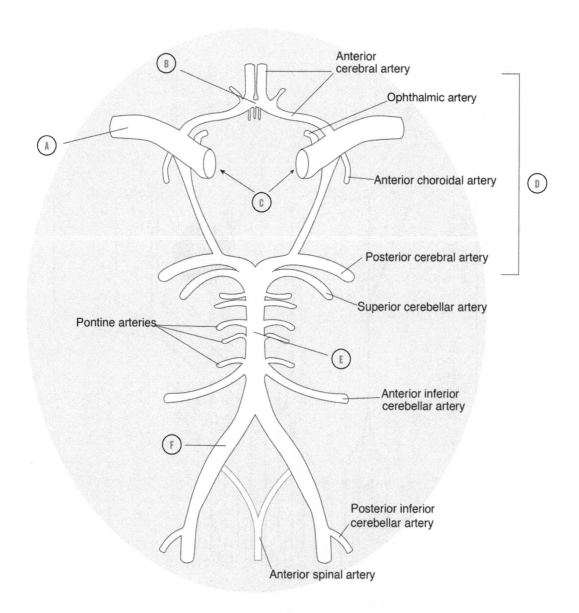

NUTRITION AND PROTECTION OF THE NERVOUS SYSTEM: CEREBROSPINAL FLUID (CSF)

INTRODUCTION

CSF protects and nourishes the central nervous system. The flow of CSF is as follows:

1. CSF is created in the choroid plexus.
2. It moves through the foramen of Monro to the third ventricle.
3. It passes through the cerebral aqueduct to the fourth ventricle.
4. It then passes through three apertures (two lateral and one median) to the cerebellomedullary cistern.
5. From here it circulates over the spinal cord and enters the subarachnoid space where it is reabsorbed.

COLOURING NOTES 5.11

- ☐ Draw arrows on the diagram to illustrate the direction of flow of CSF through the central nervous system.
- ☐ Identify and label the following:
  - ○ Third ventricle
  - ○ Fourth ventricle
  - ○ Lateral ventricle
  - ○ Subarachnoid space
  - ○ Cerebellum.
- ☐ Colour CSF filled spaces orange.
- ☐ Colour the midbrain blue.
- ☐ Colour all bones yellow.
- ☐ Colour the cerebellum purple.

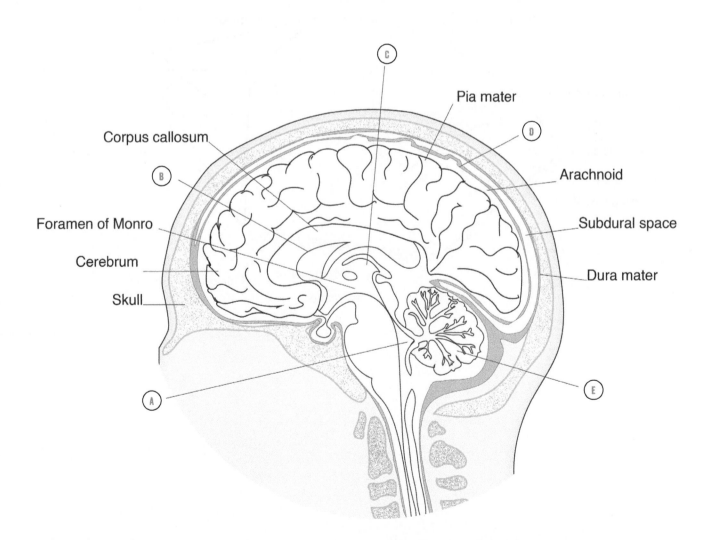

THE MENINGES

INTRODUCTION

The meninges are three layers of connective tissue that surround the brain and spinal cord: the dura, arachnoid and pia mater.

COLOURING NOTES 5.12

- ☐ Identify and label the following:
  - ○ Dura mater
  - ○ Arachnoid mater
  - ○ Pia mater
  - ○ Skull.
- ☐ Colour the dura mater orange.

- ☐ Colour the arachnoid mater blue.
- ☐ Colour the pia mater purple.
- ☐ Colour the skull grey.
- ☐ Colour the white matter yellow.
- ☐ Colour the grey matter green.

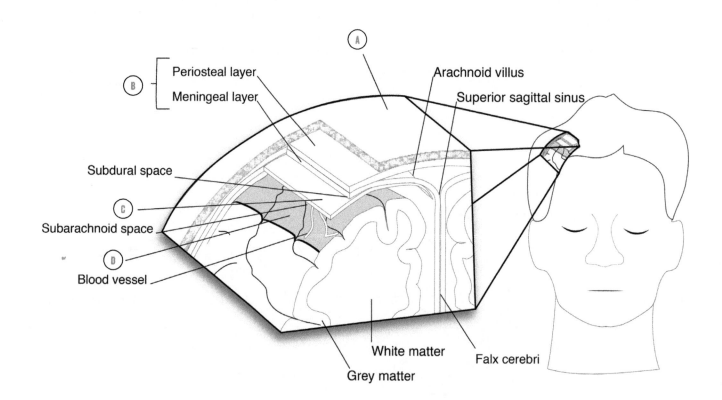

B
Periosteal layer
Meningeal layer

A

Arachnoid villus
Superior sagittal sinus

Subdural space

C

Subarachnoid space

D

Blood vessel

White matter
Grey matter
Falx cerebri

The Nurse's Anatomy and Physiology Colouring Book published 2017 by SAGE Publishing. © Jennifer Boore, Neal Cook and Andrea Shepherd.

CHAPTER 6

SPECIAL AND GENERAL SENSES: RESPONDING TO THE ENVIRONMENT

INTRODUCTION

The sensory system is fundamental to a person's relationship with their environment. Additionally, the senses are fundamental to health-related quality of life in that they enable people to derive pleasure through the experience of their environment. This chapter will help you to review the structures and functions of the special senses and the general senses. Remember to revise Chapter 6 in *Essentials of Anatomy and Physiology for Nursing Practice*.

Answers to the labelling exercises can be found at the back of the book.

COMPONENTS OF THE EYE

INTRODUCTION

The eye is a sphere about 2.5 cm in diameter and five sixths of it is concealed within the orbit, with one sixth visible. It has three principle components:

1. The three-layered wall.
2. The optical components that focus light and regulate its entry to the eye.
3. Neurological components that convert light to electrochemical energy to generate images.

COLOURING NOTES 6.1

- ☐ Identify and label the following:
  - ○ Posterior cavity
  - ○ Anterior cavity
  - ○ Ciliary body
  - ○ Optic disc
  - ○ Optic nerve
  - ○ Sclera
  - ○ Retina
  - ○ Choroid
  - ○ Cornea
  - ○ Lens
  - ○ Pupil
  - ○ Iris.
- ☐ Colour the posterior cavity light green.
- ☐ Colour the anterior cavity dark blue.
- ☐ Colour the ciliary body pink.
- ☐ Colour the optic nerve red.
- ☐ Colour the sclera yellow.
- ☐ Colour the retina orange.
- ☐ Colour the choroid dark green.
- ☐ Colour the cornea light blue.
- ☐ Colour the iris purple.

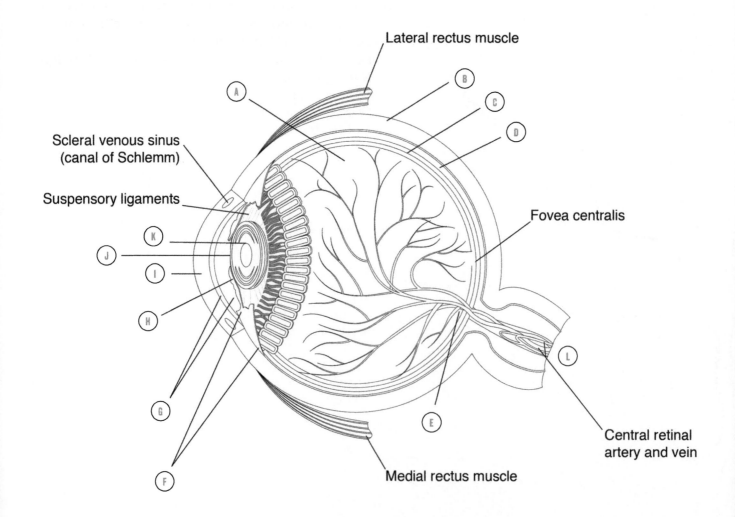

Lateral rectus muscle

Scleral venous sinus (canal of Schlemm)

Suspensory ligaments

Fovea centralis

Central retinal artery and vein

Medial rectus muscle

LIGHT REFRACTION IN THE EYE

INTRODUCTION

As light enters the eye, it is bent by the fixed surface of the cornea and then by the lens (both on entering and exiting the lens). Some 75% of refraction occurs in the cornea and is unchanging while 25% of refraction in the lens is adjustable.

COLOURING NOTES 6.2

Draw in the refraction lines from the book through the pupil into the eye and onto the retina (see p. 152 of *Essentials of Anatomy and Physiology for Nursing Practice*). Colour the refractory areas yellow.

See p. 152 of *Essentials of Anatomy and Physiology for Nursing Practice* to check the answers.

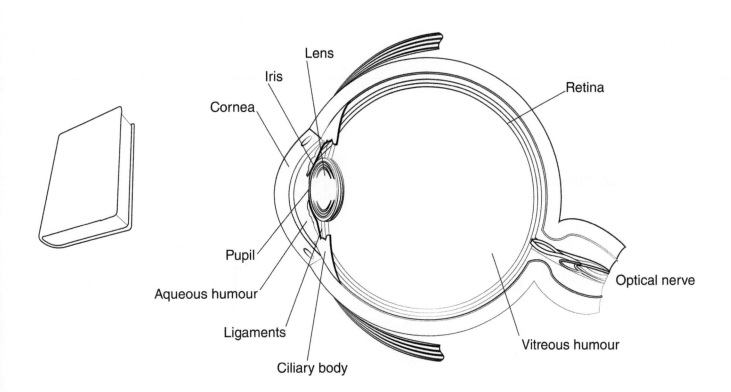

TASTE

INTRODUCTION

Gustation occurs from chemicals reacting with taste buds (of which there are about 10,000). These are primarily located on the tongue, but also on the inside surface of the cheeks and the soft palate, pharynx and epiglottis. These taste buds can distinguish five primary tastes:

- **Sweet:** Mostly stimulated by sugary carbohydrates.
- **Sour:** Stimulated mainly by acids such as fruit acids.
- **Bitter:** Primarily stimulated by alkaloids in plant leaves and food that has spoiled.
- **Salty:** triggered by metal ions, such as sodium and potassium.
- **Umami:** This is the meaty/savoury taste found in protein foods such as meat and fish (no specific zone on the tongue).

COLOURING NOTES 6.3

- ☐ Label the taste zones and papillae.
- ☐ Colour the sour zones yellow.
- ☐ Colour the salty zones orange.
- ☐ Colour the sweet zone dark blue.

- ☐ Colour the bitter zone purple.
- ☐ Colour the circumvallate papillae light blue.
- ☐ Colour the rest of the tongue red.

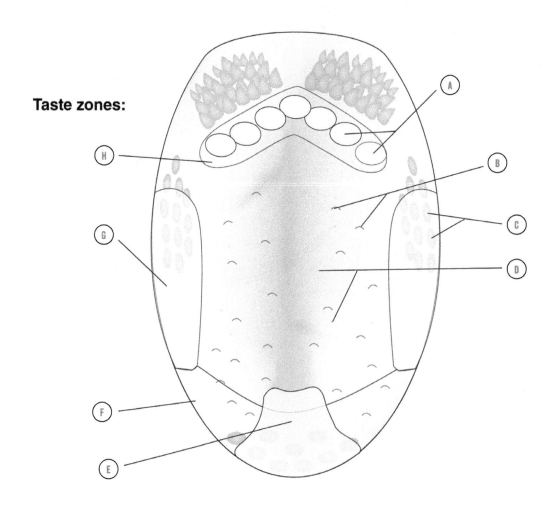

Taste zones:

TASTE BUD

INTRODUCTION

Taste buds consist of three types of cells: taste cells, supporting cells and basal cells.

COLOURING NOTES 6.4

☐ Identify and label the following:
  ○ Taste pore
  ○ Gustatory hair
  ○ Gustatory receptor cell
  ○ Supporting cell
  ○ Sensory neurons
  ○ Connective tissue
  ○ Basal cell.

☐ Colour the gustatory hair light blue.
☐ Colour the gustatory receptor cells dark blue.
☐ Colour the basal cells purple.
☐ Colour the supporting cells green.
☐ Colour the sensory neurons yellow.

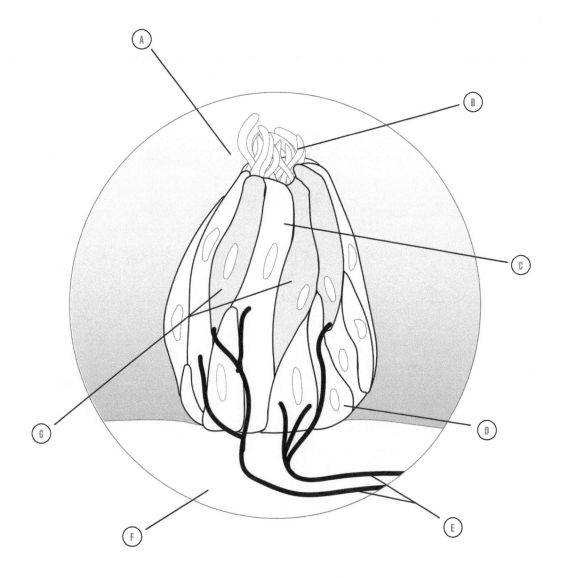

OLFACTION

INTRODUCTION

Olfaction, or smell, is the second chemical sense with the primary sense organ in the olfactory mucosa in the superior nasal cavity. Olfaction is highly sensitive, with some people able to identify up to 10,000 smells using the 10–20 million olfactory cells in the olfactory mucosa. Supporting cells provide electrical insulation, protection and nourishment to the olfactory neurons while also detoxifying chemicals, while the basal cells divide and differentiate into new olfactory neurons.

COLOURING NOTES 6.5

- ☐ Identify and label the following:
  - ○ Olfactory bulb
  - ○ Cribriform formina
  - ○ Axon
  - ○ Basal cell
  - ○ Supporting cell
  - ○ Olfactory neuron
  - ○ Dendrite
  - ○ Cilia
  - ○ Olfactory vesicle.
- ☐ Colour the olfactory tract and axons green.
- ☐ Colour the supporting cells blue.
- ☐ Colour the basal cells purple.

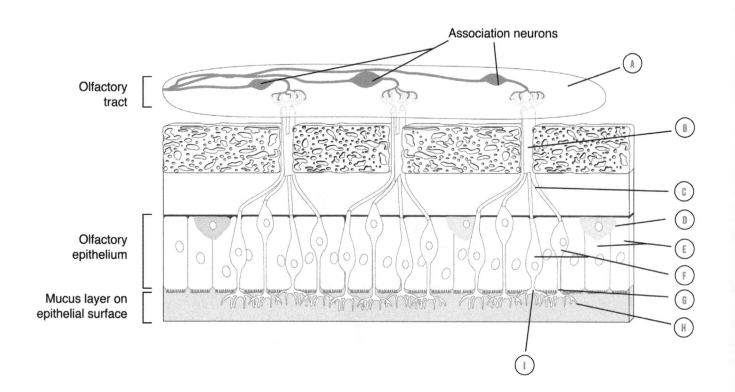

ANATOMY OF THE EAR

INTRODUCTION

The ear has the important role of funnelling sounds for sensory reception and interpretation. It also has a role in equilibrium which refers to the sense that helps maintain balance and awareness of orientation in space (proprioception). The ear is divided into three main regions:

- **External ear:** to collect sound waves and channel them inwards.
- **Middle ear:** to convey sound vibrations to the oval window and inner ear.
- **Internal (inner) ear:** to house receptors for hearing and equilibrium.

--- **COLOURING NOTES 6.6** ---

☐ Identify and label the following:

- ○ Auricle
- ○ Temporal bone
- ○ Auditory canal
- ○ Ear lobe
- ○ Tympanic membrane
- ○ Malleus
- ○ Incus
- ○ Stapes
- ○ Semi-circular canals
- ○ Oval window
- ○ Auditory tube
- ○ Cochlea.

☐ Colour the cochlea blue.
☐ Colour the oval window yellow.
☐ Colour the auditory ossicles green.
☐ Colour the tympanic membrane pink.
☐ Colour the auditory tube orange.
☐ Colour the auditory canal brown.

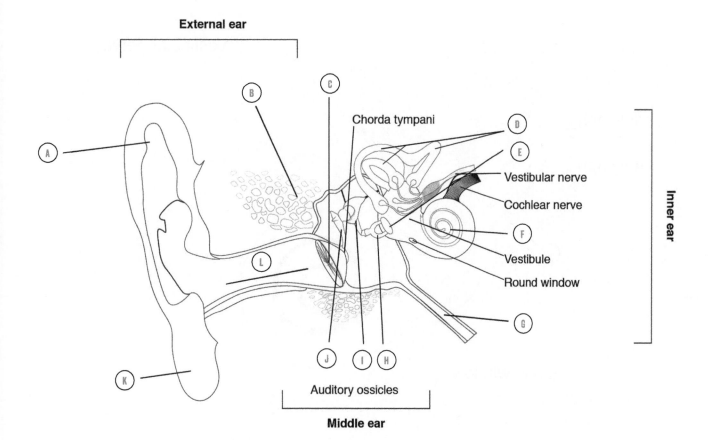

External ear

Chorda tympani

Vestibular nerve

Cochlear nerve

Vestibule

Round window

Inner ear

Auditory ossicles

Middle ear

THE VESTIBULAR APPARATUS

INTRODUCTION

The vestibular apparatus is the organ of balance. It consists of the vestibule and the semi-circular canals. The vestibule consists of a pair of membranous sacs, the saccule and utricle. Both of these contain maculae essential for maintaining appropriate posture and balance as they provide sensory information on the position of the head in space. Maculae consist of two kinds of cells: hair cells, which are the sensory receptors, and support cells, which secrete a thick gelatinous glycoprotein layer known as the otolithic membrane. The three semi-circular canals that function in dynamic equilibrium are:

- Anterior.
- Posterior.
- Lateral.

COLOURING NOTES 6.7

☐ Identify and label the following:

- ○ Semi-circular canals
- ○ Utricle
- ○ Saccule
- ○ Cochlea
- ○ Oval window

- ○ Ampulla
- ○ Auditory nerve.

☐ Colour the semi-circular canals blue.
☐ Colour the auditory nerve yellow.
☐ Colour the cochlea green.
☐ Colour the oval and round windows black.

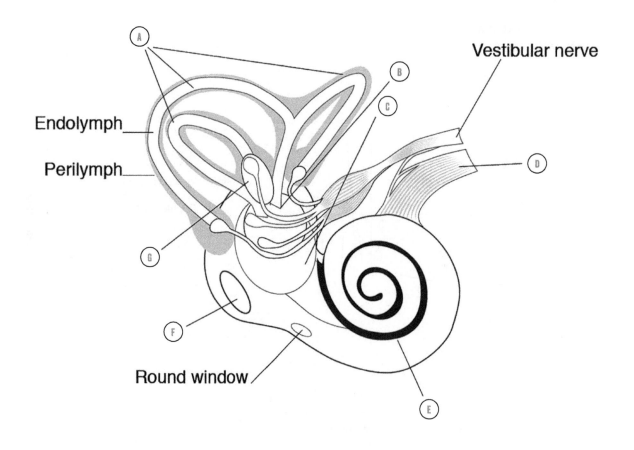

GENERAL SENSES

INTRODUCTION

The general senses refer to the sensations of pain, temperature and touch (pressure, vibration and proprioception). Their receptors' structure and physiology are largely quite simple and generally composed of a sensory nerve fibre and a small amount of connective tissue. Sensory receptors for the general senses are classified as either encapsulated or unencapsulated.

COLOURING NOTES 6.8

- ☐ Identify and label the following:
  - ○ Merkel cells
  - ○ Tactile discs
  - ○ Tactile corpuscle
  - ○ Free nerve endings
  - ○ Ruffini corpuscles

  - ○ Root hair plexus
  - ○ Lamellated corpuscles.
- ☐ Colour the tactile corpuscles blue.
- ☐ Colour the lamellated and Ruffinni corpuscles green.
- ☐ Colour the free nerve endings yellow.
- ☐ Colour the rest of the skin light brown.

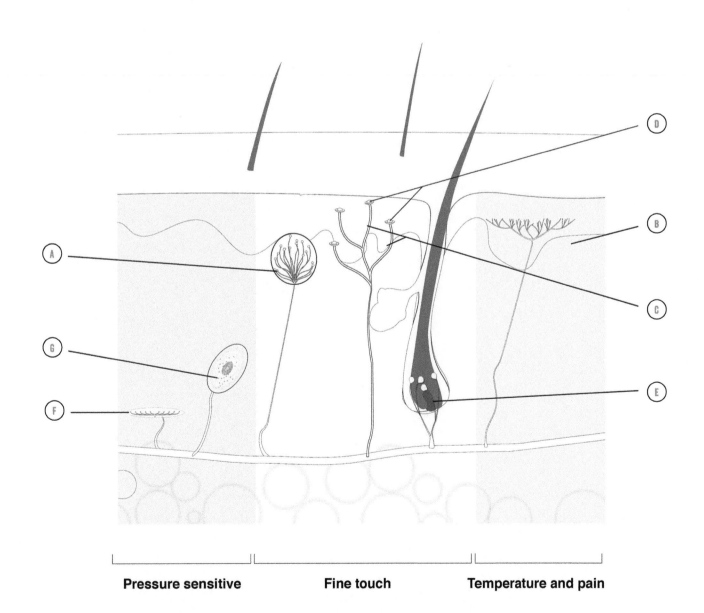

Pressure sensitive   Fine touch   Temperature and pain

CHAPTER 7

THE ENDOCRINE SYSTEM: CONTROL OF INTERNAL FUNCTIONS

INTRODUCTION

The endocrine system is of significant importance at all stages throughout life. It plays a major role in contributing to the maintenance of homeostasis, including its relationship with other systems in the body, particularly the nervous system. Hormones influence the function of glands to regulate the internal environment, including metabolism, growth and development, tissue function, sleep, and mood. This chapter will revisit the structures of the endocrine system to enable you to understand how it operates. Remember to revise Chapter 7 in *Essentials of Anatomy and Physiology for Nursing Practice*.

Answers to the labelling exercises can be found at the back of the book.

HORMONES AND THEIR MODE OF ACTION

IINTRODUCTION

Hormones link with receptors to modulate their function in the different modes of hormone action:

- Classical.
- Paracrine.
- Juxtacrine.
- Autocrine.
- Intracrine.

─────────── COLOURING NOTES 7.1 ───────────

☐ Label each of the modes of action.
☐ Draw arrows to indicate the movement of hormones towards their site of action.
☐ Colour the nucleus of each cell purple.
☐ Colour the cytoplasm of each cell yellow.

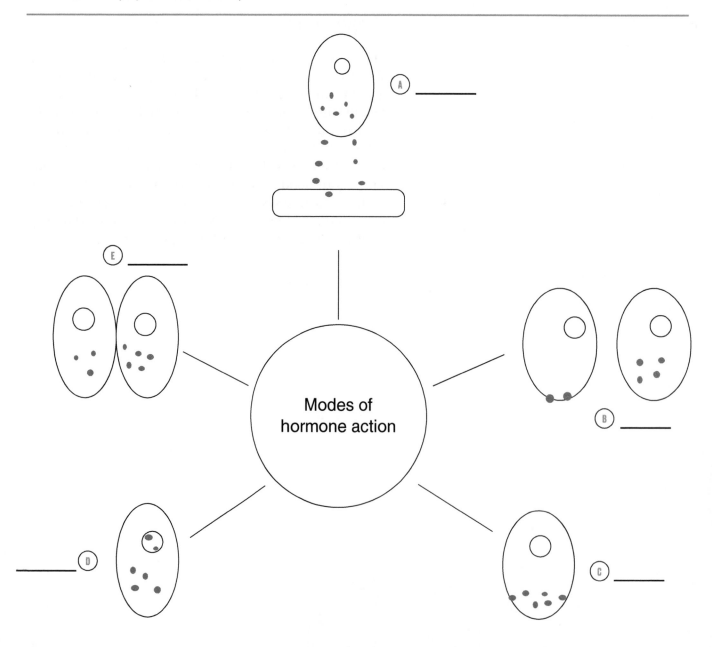

MAJOR ENDOCRINE ORGANS

INTRODUCTION

The endocrine system works alongside the nervous system to coordinate the functions of all body systems. The endocrine system works slowly and is often responsible for the regulation of longer-term processes. It does this by releasing chemical mediators known as hormones. The endocrine system is comprised of endocrine glands that include the pituitary, thyroid, parathyroid, adrenal and pineal glands and several organs and tissues that contain cells that can secrete hormones, including the hypothalamus, thymus, pancreas, ovaries, testes, kidneys, liver, stomach, small intestine, skin and heart.

—————————————————— **COLOURING NOTES 7.2** ——————————————————

☐ Identify and label the following:
- ○ Hypothalamus
- ○ Thyroid
- ○ Pituitary
- ○ Pancreas
- ○ Adrenal glands
- ○ Ovaries
- ○ Testes

- ○ Parathyroid
- ○ Pineal
- ○ Thymus.

☐ Colour the pancreas purple.
☐ Colour the adrenal glands green.
☐ Colour the thyroid blue.
☐ Colour the thymus red.

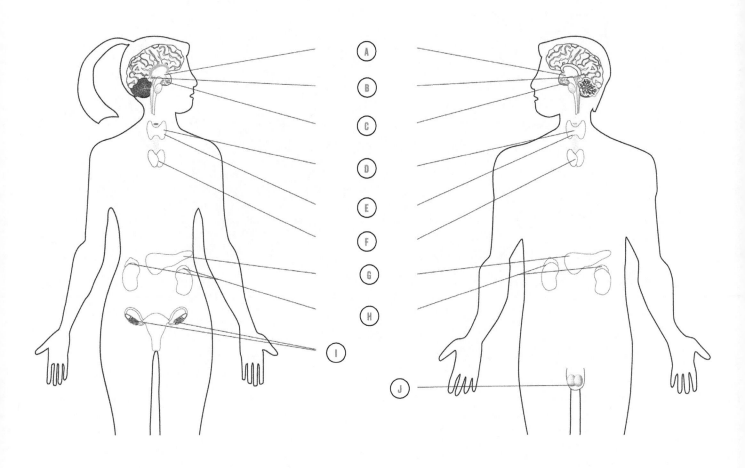

MAJOR ENDOCRINE ORGANS (CONTINUED)

─── COLOURING NOTES 7.3 ───

☐ Identify and label the following:
  ○ Hypothalamus
  ○ Pineal gland
  ○ Thalamus
  ○ Pituitary gland.

☐ Colour the hypothalamus orange.
☐ Colour the pituitary gland green.
☐ Colour the pineal gland blue.
☐ Colour the thalamus red.

COLOURING NOTES 7.4

☐ Identify and label the thyroid gland. Colour it orange.
☐ Identify and label the parathyroid glands. Colour them blue.

☐ Colour the thyroid cartilage green.
☐ Colour the rings of cartilage on the trachea yellow.

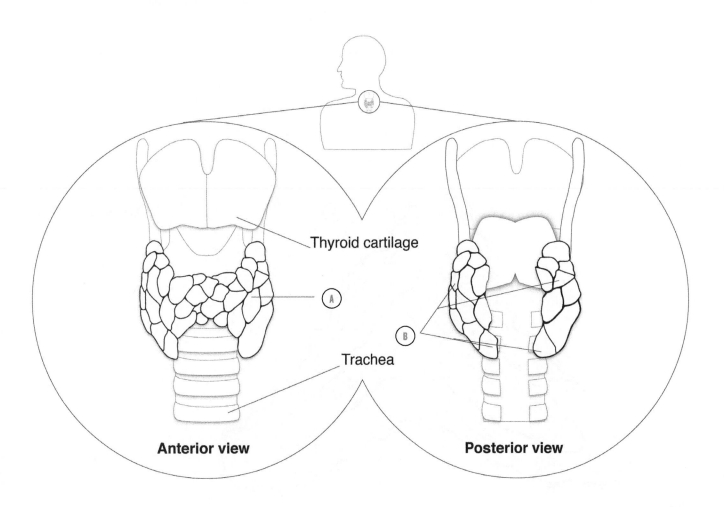

Thyroid cartilage

Ⓐ

Trachea

Ⓑ

Anterior view

Posterior view

ADRENAL GLANDS

INTRODUCTION

The two adrenal glands are positioned on the top of the kidneys and each consists of two separate parts – the cortex and the medulla both of which secrete hormones as part of maintaining homeostasis.

COLOURING NOTES 7.5

- ☐ Identify and label the following:
  - ○ Zona fasciculata
  - ○ Zona glomerulosa
  - ○ Zona reticularis
  - ○ Medulla.

- ☐ Colour the zona glomerulosa orange.
- ☐ Colour the zona fasciculatea pink.
- ☐ Colour the zona reticularis purple.
- ☐ Colour the medulla red.

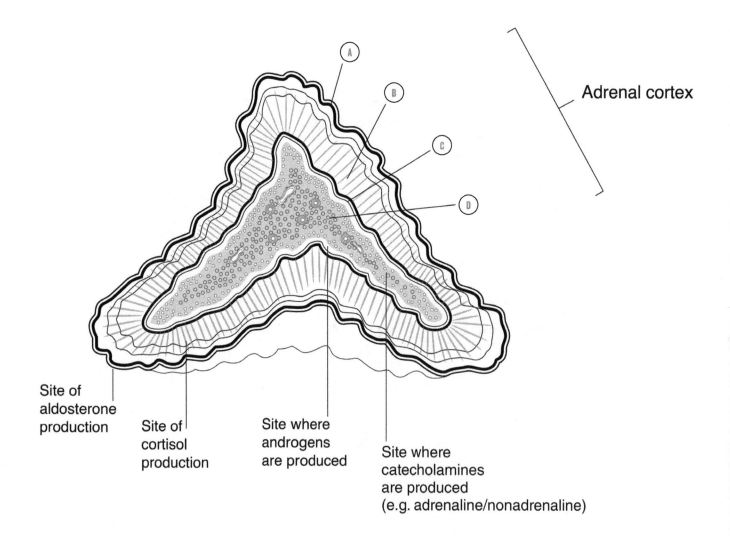

Adrenal cortex

Site of aldosterone production

Site of cortisol production

Site where androgens are produced

Site where catecholamines are produced (e.g. adrenaline/nonadrenaline)

ISLET OF LANGERHANS

INTRODUCTION

The pancreas lies in the abdomen and plays an important role in digestion as an exocrine gland secreting its enzymes into the duodenum for digestion of carbohydrates, lipids and proteins. Its endocrine function is concerned with glucose metabolism through the secretion of hormones from the specialised cells of the islets of Langerhans.

COLOURING NOTES 7.6

- ☐ Identify and label the gamma cells. Colour them yellow.
- ☐ Identify and label the alpha cells. Colour them green.
- ☐ Identify and label the blood capillaries. Colour them red.
- ☐ Identify and label the beta cells. Colour them blue.

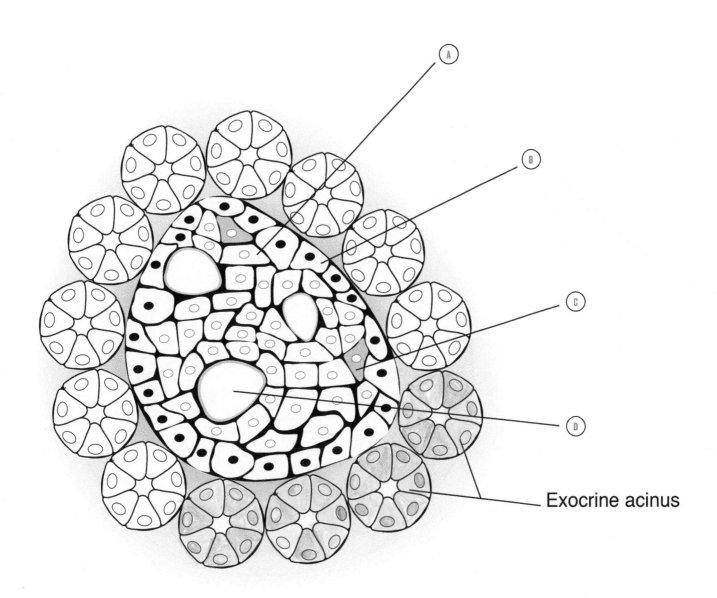

A

B

C

D

Exocrine acinus

THE RENIN ANGIOTENSIN ALDOSTERONE SYSTEM (RAAS): THE JUXTAGLOMERULAR APPARATUS

INTRODUCTION

Renin secretion is the key element in the RAAS and is regulated through the Juxtaglomerular Apparatus (JGA) (or granular cells). The macula densa is composed of specialised columnar epithelium cells which sense the concentration of sodium in the distal part of the renal tubule.

─────── COLOURING NOTES 7.7 ───────

- ☐ Identify and label the following:
  - ○ Afferent arteriole
  - ○ Macula densa cells
  - ○ Proximal tubule cells
  - ○ Efferent arteriole
  - ○ Granular cells
  - ○ Red blood cells
  - ○ Glomerular capsule.
- ☐ Colour the capsular space orange.
- ☐ Colour the afferent and efferent arterioles red.
- ☐ Colour the macula densa cells blue.
- ☐ Colour the granular cells yellow.

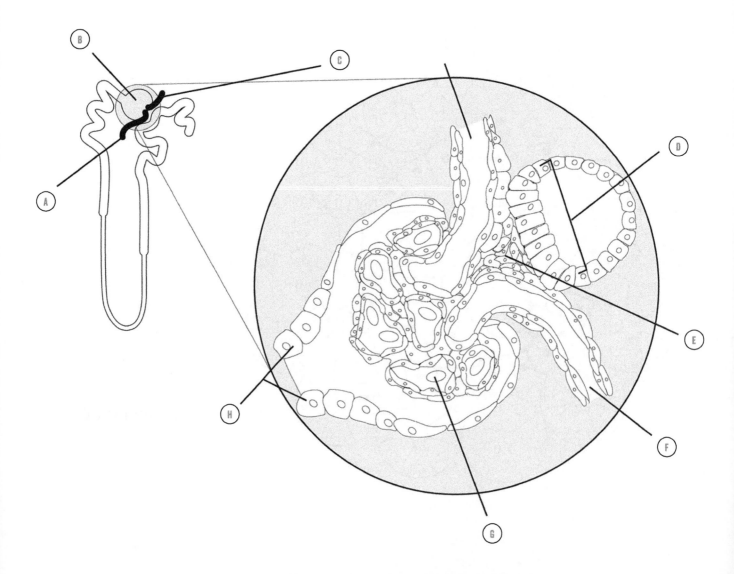

RAAS

INTRODUCTION

This is an important system in relation to fluid and electrolyte balance and blood pressure. It demonstrates the interaction between different organs in endocrine control. The liver produces the protein angiotensinogen which is converted to an active hormone (angiotensin I) by an enzyme secreted by the kidney (renin). Angiotensin Converting Enzyme (ACE), partly secreted by the lungs, converts angiotensin I to angiotensin II.

—————————————————— COLOURING NOTES 7.8 ——————————————————

Fill in the blank parts of the RAAS. Link the parts together logically with arrows.

See p. 189 of *Essentials of Anatomy and Physiology for Nursing Practice* to check the answers.

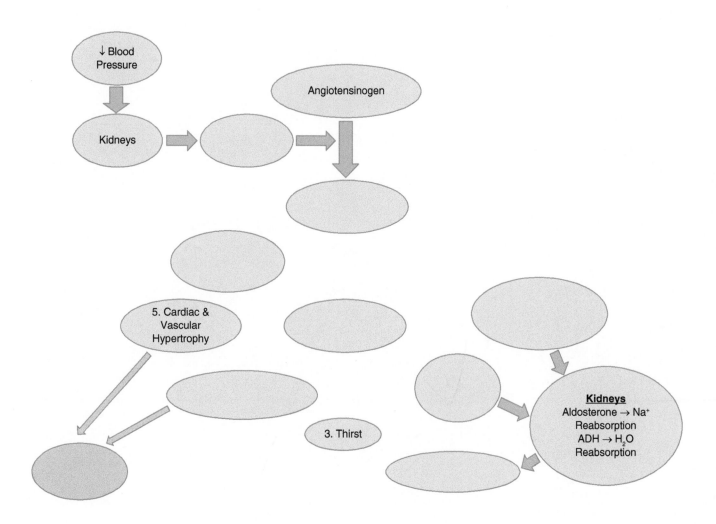

CHAPTER 8

THE DIGESTIVE SYSTEM: NUTRIENT SUPPLY AND WASTE ELIMINATION

INTRODUCTION

The digestive system represents a vital link between the external and internal environments. Its contribution to homeostasis is through the provision of nutrients to the internal environment and the removal of waste products. This chapter will revisit the structure of the components of the digestive system. It will also help you to refresh your knowledge on how the digestive system contributes to homeostasis. Remember to revise Chapter 8 in *Essentials of Anatomy and Physiology for Nursing Practice*.

Answers to the labelling exercises can be found at the back of the book.

COMPONENTS OF THE DIGESTIVE SYSTEM

INTRODUCTION

Technically, the digestive tract is outside the body and therefore part of the external environment: it is essentially a tube through the body with the purpose of moving nutrients from the external environment into the internal environment. The digestive tract runs through the body from the mouth to the anus, supported in its role by a number of accessory organs.

COLOURING NOTES 8.1

- ☐ Identify and label the pancreas. Colour it dark green.
- ☐ Identify and label the gall bladder. Colour it light green.
- ☐ Identify and label the small intestine. Colour it orange.
- ☐ Identify and label the large intestine. Colour it brown.
- ☐ Identify and label the liver. Colour it purple.
- ☐ Identify and label the stomach. Colour it red.
- ☐ Identify and label the oesophagus. Colour it blue.

- ☐ Identify and label the rectum. Colour it yellow.
- ☐ Identify and label the mouth. Colour it pink.
- ☐ Identify and label the following:
  - ○ Duodenum
  - ○ Beginning of large intestine
  - ○ End of small intestine
  - ○ Anus.

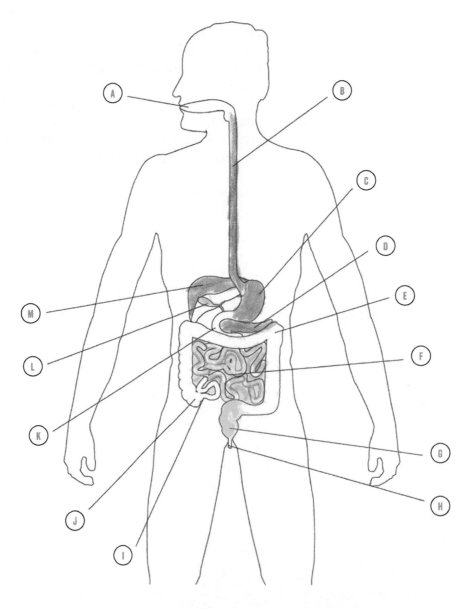

STRUCTURE OF THE DIGESTIVE TRACT

INTRODUCTION

Tubular structures are muscular, enabling them to move contents within and through them, and the digestive tract uses this movement to mechanically digest (i.e. break down into smaller particles) and propel contents along its length.

COLOURING NOTES 8.2

☐ Identify and label the circular layer. Colour it red.
☐ Identify and label the epithelium. Colour it pink.
☐ Identify and label the lamina propria. Colour it purple.
☐ Identify and label the mesentery. Colour it brown.
☐ Identify and label the muscularis mucosa. Colour it blue.
☐ Identify and label the outer longitudinal layer. Colour it green.

☐ Identify and label the serosa. Colour it orange.
☐ Identify and label the submucosa. Colour it yellow.
☐ Identify and label the following:
 ○ Artery
 ○ Lymph vessel
 ○ Vein
 ○ Villi.

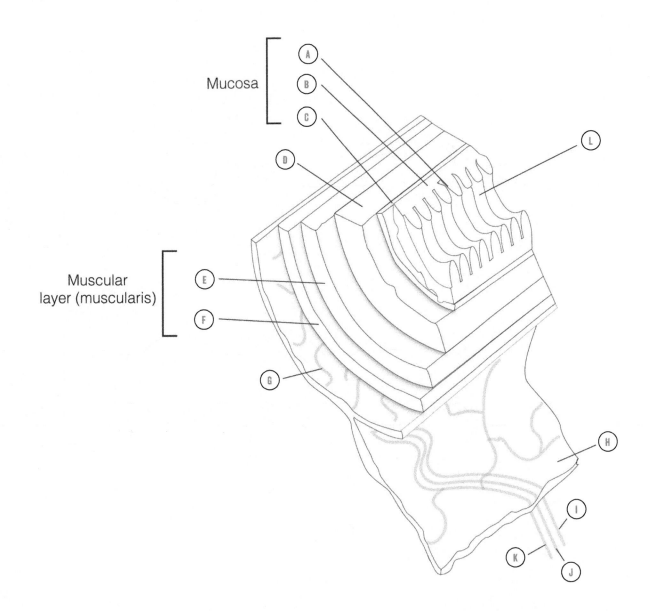

The Nurse's Anatomy and Physiology Colouring Book published 2017 by SAGE Publishing. © Jennifer Boore, Neal Cook and Andrea Shepherd.

MOVEMENTS OF THE GUT

INTRODUCTION

The two types of movement in the gut are peristalsis and segmentation. Peristalsis describes ripple-like waves created by the relaxation and contraction of muscle along the entire digestive tract. This results in the movement of material along the digestive tract. Segmentation mixes the contents of the gut, i.e. food and digestive enzymes to promote digestion.

--- COLOURING NOTES 8.3 ---

☐ Identify the food bolus. Colour it orange.
☐ Identify the points of contraction in each image.
☐ Using arrows, show the direction of movement of the food bolus in both images.
☐ Identify and label which of the images represent peristaltic movement and segmentation movement.

See p. 214 of *Essentials of Anatomy and Physiology for Nursing Practice* to check the answers.

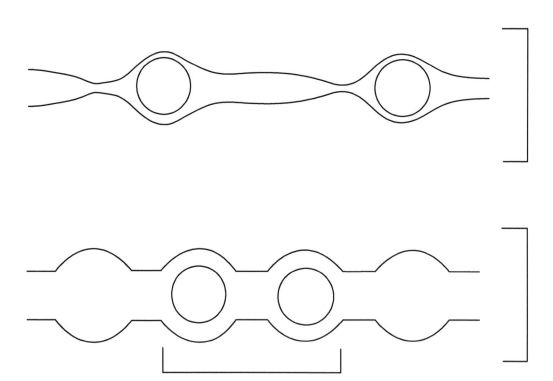

TOOTH ANATOMY

INTRODUCTION

Teeth are designed for biting, chewing (mastication) and grinding food when the upper and lower teeth are moved against each other by the muscular movement of the mandible (jaw). Teeth are composed of four primary layers:

- Enamel.
- Dentine.
- Cementum.
- Pulp.

COLOURING NOTES 8.4

- ☐ Identify and label the bone. Colour it orange.
- ☐ Identify and label the dentine. Colour it blue.
- ☐ Identify and label the enamel. Colour it yellow.
- ☐ Identify and label the gums. Colour them red.
- ☐ Identify and label the pulp. Colour it purple.

- ☐ Identify and label the following:
  - ○ Cementum
  - ○ Crown
  - ○ Nerves and blood vessels
  - ○ Root end opening.

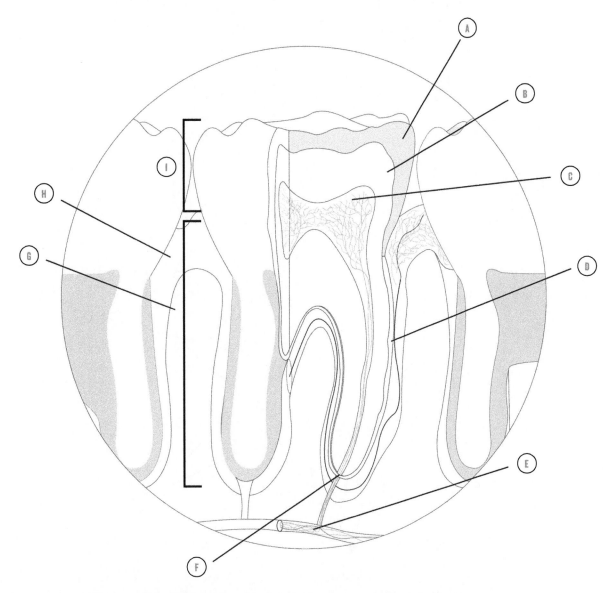

TYPES AND LOCATION OF TEETH

INTRODUCTION

People have two sets of teeth. The first 20 (deciduous or primary teeth) appear in the first two years of life. The 32 permanent teeth emerge and begin replacing primary teeth from approximately the age of six, taking up to the age of 25 to complete. There are four types of teeth:

- Incisors.
- Canines.
- Premolars.
- Molars.

COLOURING NOTES 8.5

☐ Identify and label a canine. Colour the canines yellow.
☐ Identify and label the incisors. Colour them blue.
☐ Identify and label the molars. Colour them pink.
☐ Identify and label the premolars. Colour them green.

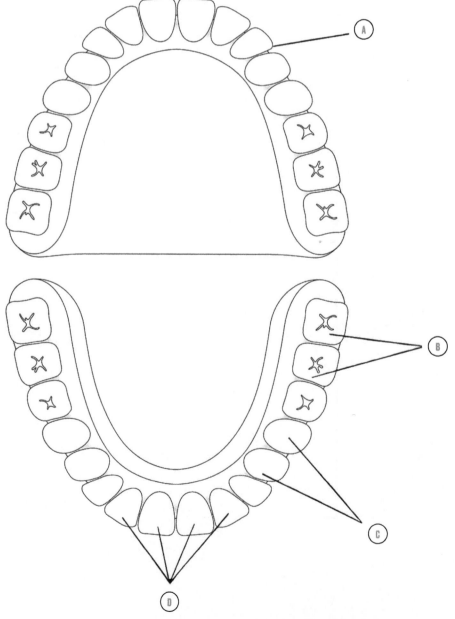

SALIVARY GLANDS AND DUCTS

INTRODUCTION

Opening into the mouth are three pairs of salivary glands: parotid, submandibular and sublingual. These produce and secrete saliva, a slightly acidic liquid, into the mouth through ducts.

--- **COLOURING NOTES 8.6** ---

☐ Identify and label the parotid glands. Colour them blue.
☐ Identify and label the sublingual glands. Colour them green.
☐ Identify and label the submandibular glands. Colour them yellow.

☐ Identify and label the following:
  ○ Parotid ducts
  ○ Sublingual duct
  ○ Submandibular duct.

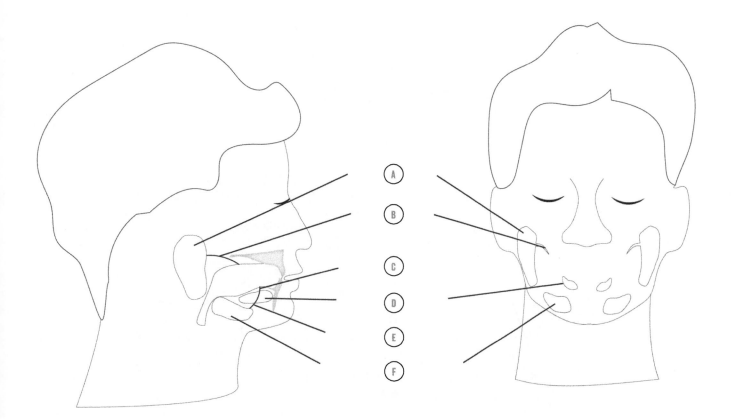

PARTS OF THE STOMACH

INTRODUCTION

The stomach is a bean-shaped sac designed to house food for digestion. As the food bolus moves into the stomach, the pyloric sphincter (at the exit from the stomach) closes to retain the food for digestion. Chemical and mechanical digestion both occur in the stomach.

COLOURING NOTES 8.7

☐ Identify and label the following:
  ○ Body
  ○ Cardiac sphincter
  ○ Fundus
  ○ Pyloric antrum
  ○ Pyloric sphincter
  ○ Rugae.

☐ Identify and label the circular muscle. Colour it yellow.
☐ Identify and label the duodenum. Colour it purple.
☐ Identify and label the longitudinal muscle. Colour it orange.
☐ Identify and label the oblique muscle. Colour it red.
☐ Identify and label the oesophagus. Colour it blue.
☐ Identify the epithelial layer. Colour it green.
☐ Identify the serosa layer. Colour it pink.

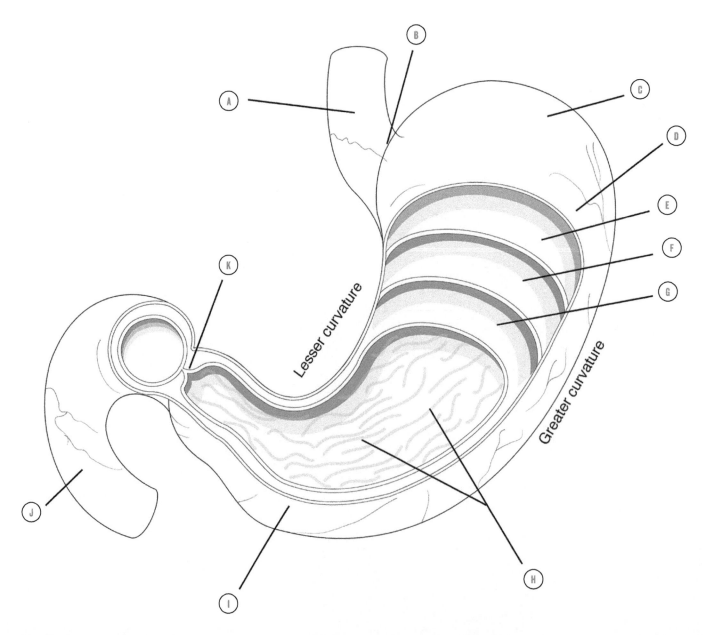

VILLI OF THE SMALL INTESTINE

INTRODUCTION

The small intestinal structure is modified to maximise absorption, with the mucosal wall structured into villi, and microvilli (also known as the brush border), increasing the surface area for absorption and also producing some enzymes. It is at the surface of microvilli that final digestion occurs through the action of brush border enzymes.

——————— COLOURING NOTES 8.8 ———————

- ☐ Identify and label the intestinal glands.
- ☐ Identify and label the villi. Colour them pink.
- ☐ Colour the vein blue.

- ☐ Colour the artery red.
- ☐ Identify and label the lacteal. Colour the lymph vessel and lacteal yellow.

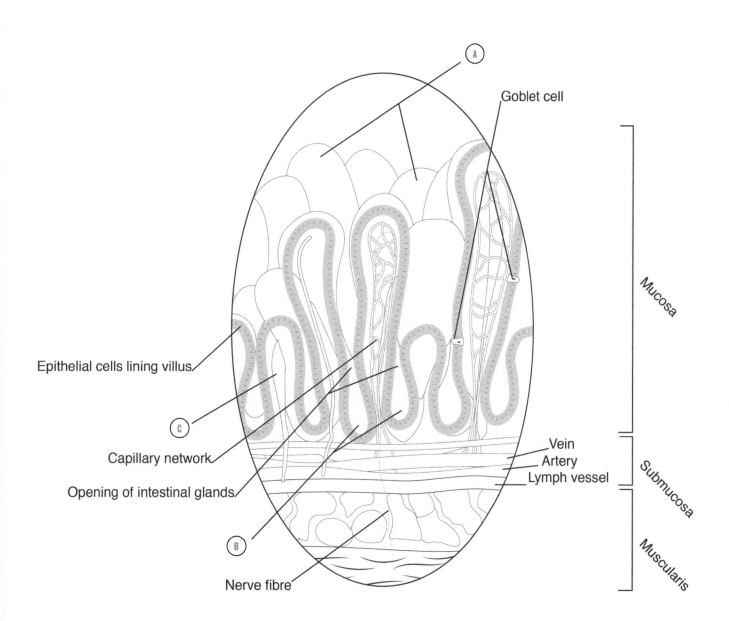

Goblet cell

Epithelial cells lining villus

Capillary network

Opening of intestinal glands

Nerve fibre

Vein
Artery
Lymph vessel

Mucosa

Submucosa

Muscularis

COMPONENTS OF THE LARGE INTESTINE

INTRODUCTION

The large intestine is laid out in a clockwise manner, with the ascending colon on the right-hand side of the body. This becomes the transverse colon, going from right to left across the body. This becomes the descending colon on the left-hand side which then extends centrally into the sigmoid colon. At the terminal end of the large intestine is the rectum which stores faeces until elimination through the anus.

COLOURING NOTES 8.9

- ☐ Identify and label the caecum and anus.
- ☐ Identify and label the vermiform appendix. Colour it red.
- ☐ Identify and label the ascending colon. Colour it orange.
- ☐ Identify and label the transverse colon. Colour it yellow.

- ☐ Identify and label the descending colon. Colour it green.
- ☐ Identify and label the sigmoid colon. Colour it blue.
- ☐ Identify and label the rectum. Colour it purple.
- ☐ Using arrows, indicate the direction of movement of chyme through the large intestine.

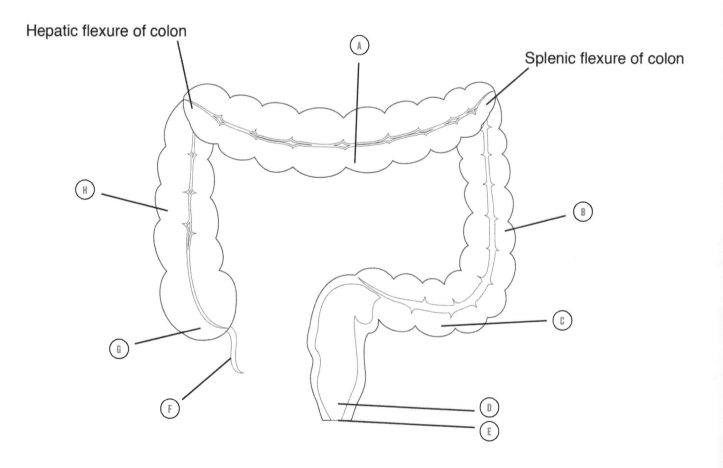

Hepatic flexure of colon

Splenic flexure of colon

CHAPTER 9

METABOLISM AND LIVER FUNCTION

INTRODUCTION

Metabolism is a series of chemical reactions that occur in the body to maintain life. The liver plays an important role in metabolism and also undertakes a number of additional functions. This chapter will help you to revise the structure of the liver and how nutrients move through the body for metabolism. You will also revisit the structure of adenosine triphosphate (ATP), the unit of energy in the body. Remember to revise Chapter 9 in *Essentials of Anatomy and Physiology for Nursing Practice*.

Answers to the labelling exercises can be found at the back of the book.

GROSS ANATOMY OF THE LIVER

INTRODUCTION

The liver is the largest glandular organ in the body and normally weighs between 1.4 and 1.6 kg in the healthy adult. It is in the right upper quadrant of the abdomen (right hypochondrium) under the diaphragm, behind and protected by the lower ribs. Gross anatomy divides the liver into four lobes based on surface features. When you look at the liver from the front (anterior surface) you will see the falciform ligament; this divides the liver into the left lobe and the right lobe (larger of the two). If the liver is flipped over to look at it from behind (posterior surface) you will see two more lobes between the right and left lobes; these are the caudate lobe (superior of the two) and the quadrate lobe.

── COLOURING NOTES 9.1 ──

Anterior view:
☐ Identify and label the falciform ligament. Colour it yellow.
☐ Identify and label the gall bladder. Colour it green.
☐ Identify and label the right and left lobes. Colour them red.

Posterior view:
☐ Identify and label the gall bladder. Colour it green.
☐ Identify and label the right, left, caudate and quadrate lobes. Colour the right red, the left orange, the caudate pink and the quadrate brown.

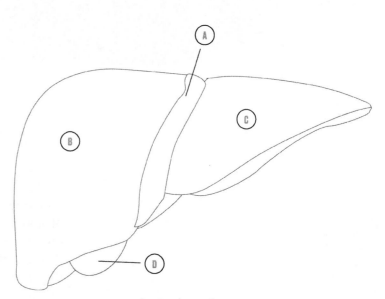

Anterior view

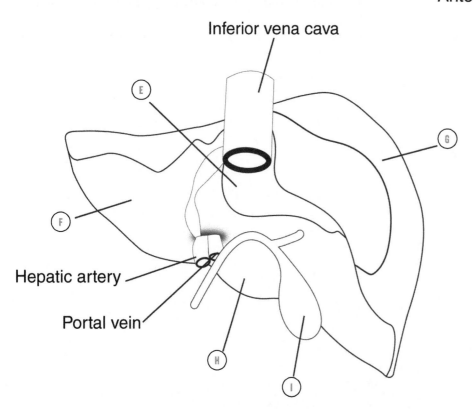

Posterior view

LIVER LOBULE

INTRODUCTION

Each lobe of the liver is made up of lobules (subdivision of a lobe). Each lobule (hexagonal in shape) consists of sheets of hepatocytes (functional cells of the liver). Each lobule is organised around a core cluster of vessels (portal triad), i.e. a branch of the hepatic artery, a branch of the portal vein and a small bile duct. The cells are arranged in pairs of columns. Between two pairs of columns of cells are sinusoids (blood vessels whose walls are incomplete). Sinusoids are lined with highly permeable endothelium which enhances transportation of nutrients into the hepatocytes.

COLOURING NOTES 9.2

☐ Identify and label a hepatocyte. Colour all the hepatocytes green.

☐ Identify and label the central vein. Colour it blue.

☐ Identify and label an interlobular vein. Colour all the interlobular veins purple.

☐ Identify and label the hepatic sinusoid.

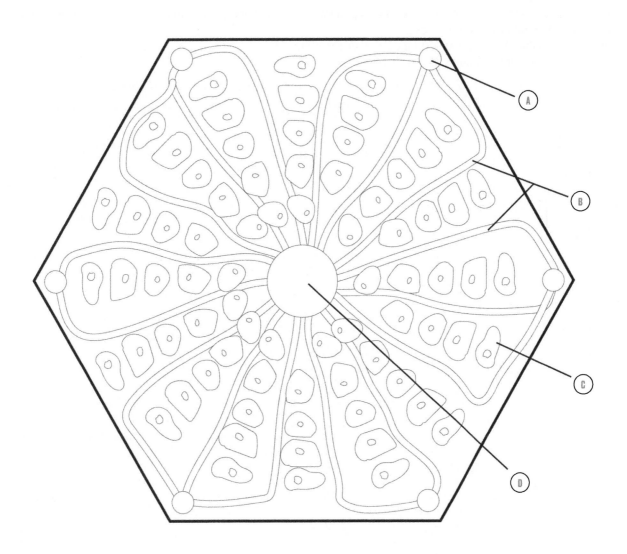

BLOOD SUPPLY TO THE LIVER

INTRODUCTION

The liver is highly vascular receiving approximately 1,600 ml (25% of cardiac output) of blood every minute, receiving this blood supply from two vessels:

- The hepatic artery (25%).
- The portal vein (75%).

The hepatic artery branches from the coeliac artery (first branch of the abdominal aorta) and delivers a rich supply of oxygenated blood to the liver cells to ensure it is well perfused to carry out its metabolic functions.

COLOURING NOTES 9.3

- ☐ Identify and colour the gall bladder green.
- ☐ Identify and label the hepatic artery and the aorta. Colour them red. Using arrows, indicate the direction of blood flow through these.
- ☐ Identify and label the hepatic vein, portal vein and inferior vena cava. Colour them blue. Using arrows, indicate the direction of blood flow through these.
- ☐ Identify and label the right and left lobes. Colour them purple.
- ☐ Identify the falciform ligament. Colour it yellow.

See p. 234 of *Essentials of Anatomy and Physiology for Nursing Practice* to check the answers.

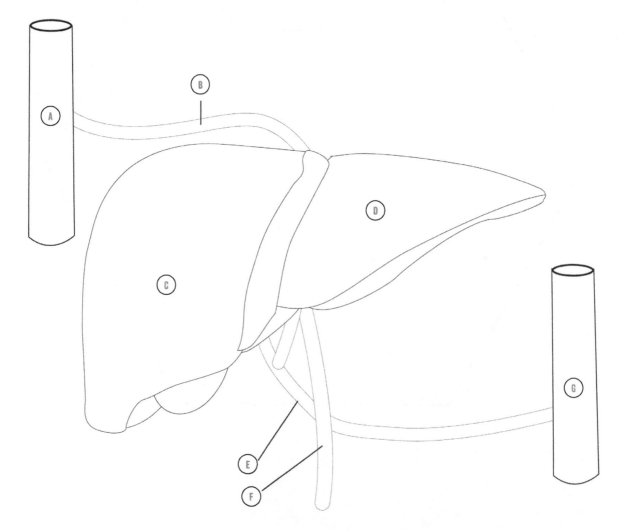

STRUCTURE OF ATP

INTRODUCTION

Adenosine triphosphate (ATP) is the key energy currency in living beings, and the formation and utilisation of ATP are generally in balance. ATP is created through a chemical cycle where adenosine diphosphate (ADP) is converted to ATP by the addition of a phosphate group linked by a high-energy bond.

--- **COLOURING NOTES 9.4** ---

☐ Colour the adenine and ribose segments pink.
☐ Colour the three phosphate group segments yellow.
☐ Draw a blue circle around the segments that together make adenosine diphosphate.
☐ Draw a circle in black to indicate the two locations of high energy bonds.
☐ Draw a green circle around the segments that together make adenosine triphosphate.
☐ Draw an orange circle around the segments that together make adenosine.

See p. 242 of *Essentials of Anatomy and Physiology for Nursing Practice* to check the answers.

Adenine (base)	Ribose (sugar)	Phosphate group	Phosphate group	Phosphate group

CHAPTER 10

THE RESPIRATORY SYSTEM: GASEOUS EXCHANGE

INTRODUCTION

Every cell in the body requires a constant supply of oxygen to undertake their metabolic functions; in doing so they produce carbon dioxide (a waste product) that must be removed. If not removed, carbon dioxide can be toxic to the cells and affect their ability to carry out their functions, thereby disturbing homeostasis. The respiratory system works hand in hand with the cardiovascular system to maintain homeostasis; the respiratory system draws oxygen from the atmosphere and expels carbon dioxide from the body, while the cardiovascular system transports the blood carrying oxygen to the cells and carbon dioxide out of the cells. This chapter will help you to review the structures of the respiratory system and how they work to support homeostasis. Remember to revise Chapter 10 in *Essentials of Anatomy and Physiology for Nursing Practice.*

Answers to the labelling exercises can be found at the back of the book.

ORGANS OF THE RESPIRATORY SYSTEM

INTRODUCTION

Structurally the respiratory system is divided into the upper respiratory tract and the lower respiratory tract. It can also be classified functionally into two distinct areas, i.e. conducting zone (carrying gases) and respiratory zone (gaseous exchange). The organs of the respiratory system are: the nose, pharynx, larynx, trachea, two bronchi, bronchioles, two lungs and muscles of breathing, i.e. the intercostal muscles and the diaphragm.

COLOURING NOTES 10.1

- ☐ Identify and label the alveoli. Colour them pink.
- ☐ Identify and label the bronchi and bronchioles. Colour them blue.
- ☐ Identify and label the diaphragm. Colour it orange.
- ☐ Identify and label the heart. Colour it red.
- ☐ Identify and label the intercostal muscles. Colour them brown.
- ☐ Identify and label the larynx. Colour it light green.
- ☐ Identify and label the nasal cavities. Colour them grey.

- ☐ Identify and label the oesophagus. Colour it dark green.
- ☐ Identify and label the pharynx. Colour it yellow.
- ☐ Identify and label the trachea. Colour it purple.
- ☐ Identify and label the following:
  - ○ Epiglottis
  - ○ Pleural membrane
  - ○ Pulmonary vessels.

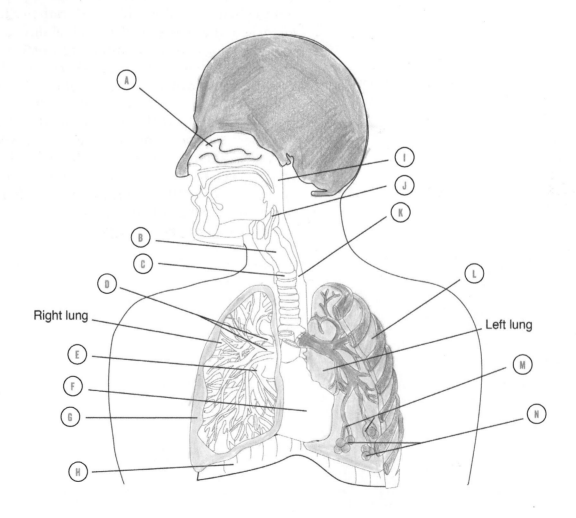

Right lung

Left lung

UPPER RESPIRATORY TRACT

INTRODUCTION

Air enters and exits the body through the upper respiratory tract. It is made up of the nose, pharynx and the larynx. It is at the point of the larynx that the upper respiratory tract ends.

COLOURING NOTES 10.2

- ☐ Identify and label the oral cavity. Colour it yellow.
- ☐ Identify and label the frontal and sphenoidal sinuses. Colour them orange.
- ☐ Identify and label the hard palate. Colour it grey.
- ☐ Identify and label the nasopharynx, oropharynx and laryngopharynx. Colour them all light blue.
- ☐ Identify and label the oesophagus. Colour it red.
- ☐ Identify and label the palatine and lingual tonsils. Colour them green.

- ☐ Identify and label the tongue. Colour it purple.
- ☐ Identify and label the trachea. Colour it dark blue.
- ☐ Identify and label the uvula. Colour it pink.
- ☐ Identify and label the following:
  - ○ Nostril
  - ○ Epiglottis.

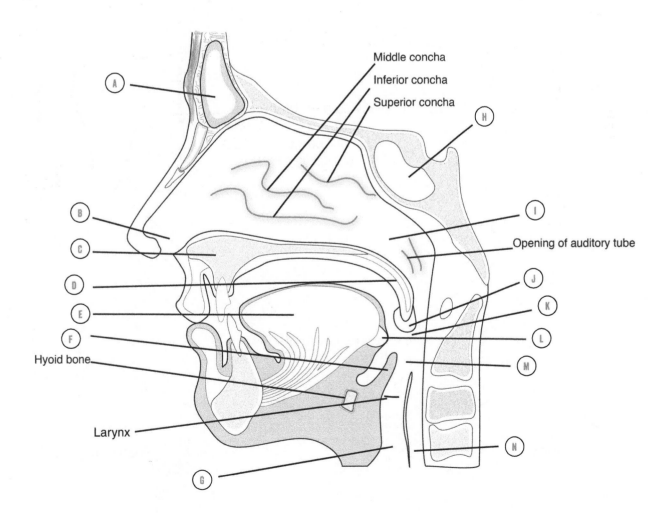

ANATOMY OF THE LARYNX

INTRODUCTION

The larynx (voice box) connects the laryngopharynx and trachea; it is positioned midline in the neck, anterior to the oesophagus and from the fourth to sixth cervical vertebrae (C4–C6). The wall of the larynx is comprised of nine pieces of cartilage; three occur singly (thyroid, cricoid and epiglottis) with the other six occurring in pairs (arytenoid, corniculate and cuneiform). The cartilages are connected to one another by muscles and ligaments; extrinsic muscles connect the cartilages to other structures in the throat, and intrinsic muscles connect the cartilages to each other.

COLOURING NOTES 10.3

- ☐ Colour the hyoid bone grey.
- ☐ Colour the thyrohyoid membrane red.
- ☐ Identify and label the arytenoid cartilage. Colour it yellow.
- ☐ Identify and label the corniculate cartilage. Colour it orange.
- ☐ Identify and label the cricoid cartilage. Colour it brown.

- ☐ Identify and label the cricothyroid ligament. Colour it black.
- ☐ Identify and label the cuneiform cartilage. Colour it blue.
- ☐ Identify and label the epiglottis. Colour it green.
- ☐ Identify and label the thyroid cartilage. Colour it purple.
- ☐ Label the trachea. Identify the c-shaped rings of hyaline cartilage around the trachea. Colour them pink.

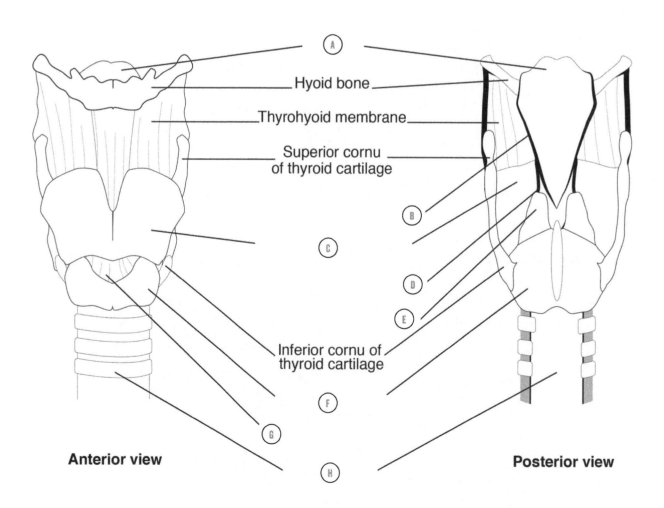

Anterior view

Posterior view

A

Hyoid bone

Thyrohyoid membrane

Superior cornu of thyroid cartilage

B

C

D

E

Inferior cornu of thyroid cartilage

F

G

H

ANATOMY OF THE BRONCHIAL TREE

INTRODUCTION

The bronchial tree is a highly branched system of conducting passages that extends from the primary bronchus to the terminal bronchioles. The trachea bifurcates into the right and left primary bronchi. The right primary bronchus is larger in diameter and extends in a more vertical direction than the left. The right primary bronchus subdivides into three secondary (lobar) bronchi and the left primary bronchus subdivides into two secondary (lobar) bronchi. The secondary bronchi then divide into the tertiary (segmental) bronchi – ten in the right lung and eight in the left.

COLOURING NOTES 10.4

- ☐ Colour the left lung tissues pink.
- ☐ Identify and label a primary bronchus. Colour both primary bronchi purple.
- ☐ Identify and label a secondary bronchus. Colour all secondary bronchi blue.
- ☐ Identify and label the trachea. Colour it red.

- ☐ Identify the lower right lung lobe. Colour it green.
- ☐ Identify the middle right lung lobe. Colour it orange.
- ☐ Identify the upper right lung lobe. Colour it yellow.
- ☐ Identify and label the following:
  - ○ Tertiary bronchi
  - ○ Bronchioles.

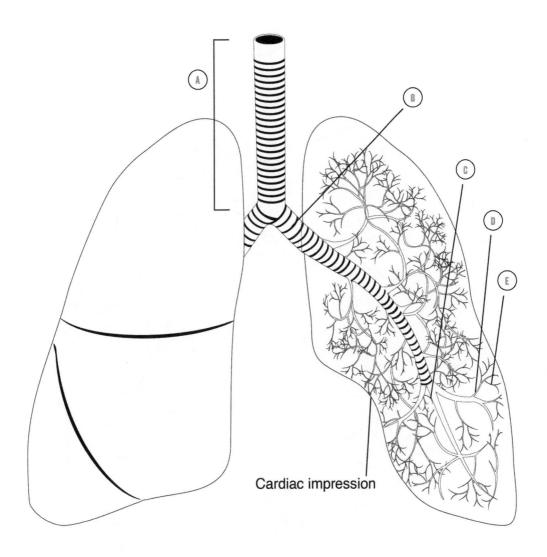

Cardiac impression

ALVEOLI

INTRODUCTION

Each adult lung consists of approximately 150 million alveoli which provide 70 m² of surface area for gaseous exchange to take place. An alveolus is a small cup-shaped pouch lined with simple squamous epithelium and supported by a thin elastic basement membrane.

COLOURING NOTES 10.5

☐ Identify and label the respiratory bronchiole. Colour it grey.

☐ Identify and label the vessel carrying deoxygenated blood from the pulmonary artery. Colour it blue.

☐ Identify and label a capillary.

☐ Identify and label the vessel carrying oxygenated blood to the pulmonary vein. Colour it red.

☐ Identify and label an alveolus. Colour the alveoli pink.

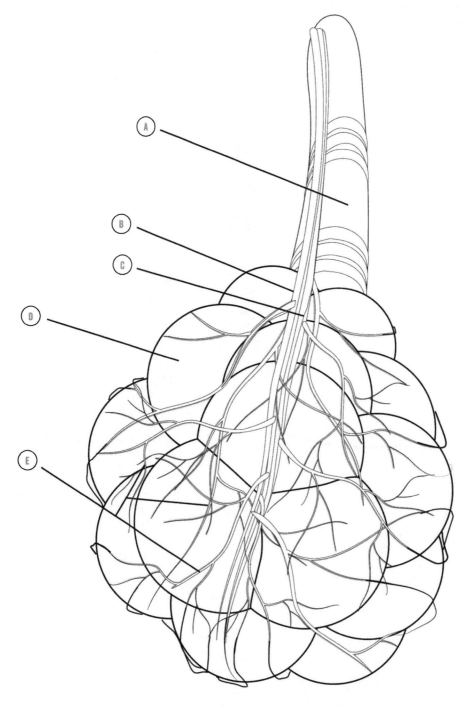

ACCESSORY MUSCLES OF RESPIRATION

INTRODUCTION

Accessory muscles of respiration are muscles that assist the diaphragm and intercostal muscles in breathing. They are used during exercise or when there is an increased effort needed for breathing, such as in some respiratory disorders.

COLOURING NOTES 10.6

- ☐ Identify and label the diaphragm. Colour it yellow.
- ☐ Identify and label the expiratory abdominal muscles. Colour them green.
- ☐ Identify and label the expiratory intercostal muscles. Colour them purple.
- ☐ Identify and label the external oblique muscles. Colour them blue.

- ☐ Identify and label the inspiratory intercostal muscles. Colour them orange.
- ☐ Identify and label the pectoralis minor. Colour them red.
- ☐ Identify and label the scalene muscles. Colour them pink.
- ☐ Identify and label the sternomastoid muscles. Colour them brown.
- ☐ Colour the bones grey.

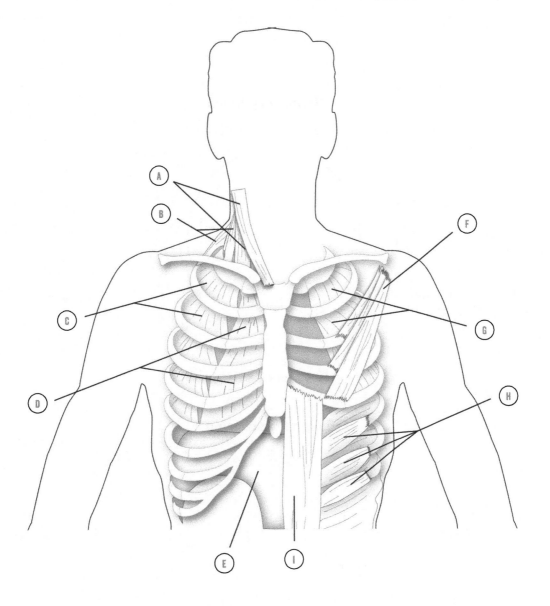

The Nurse's Anatomy and Physiology Colouring Book published 2017 by SAGE Publishing. © Jennifer Boore, Neal Cook and Andrea Shepherd.

EXTERNAL AND INTERNAL RESPIRATION

INTRODUCTION

Oxygen and carbon dioxide move between the alveolar air and pulmonary circulation through the process of passive diffusion. This is called gaseous exchange and it occurs between the alveoli and the blood (external respiration) and between the blood and cells of the body (internal respiration).

COLOURING NOTES 10.7

☐ Draw arrows to indicate the movement of gases beside the labels Inhaled O_2 and Exhaled CO_2.
☐ Draw arrows within the alveolar capillary to show the direction of blood flow.
☐ Using arrows, indicate the direction of movement of CO_2 and O_2 between the capillary and alveolus.
☐ Colour the alveolar wall pink.
☐ Identify and label the red blood cells. Colour them red.

☐ Colour the inside of the alveolus light blue.
☐ Identify and label the tissue cells. Colour them green.
☐ Using arrows, indicate the direction of movement of CO_2 and O_2 between the capillary and the tissue.
☐ Colour the intracellular fluid yellow.

See p. 277 of *Essentials of Anatomy and Physiology for Nursing Practice* to check the answers.

Internal respiration

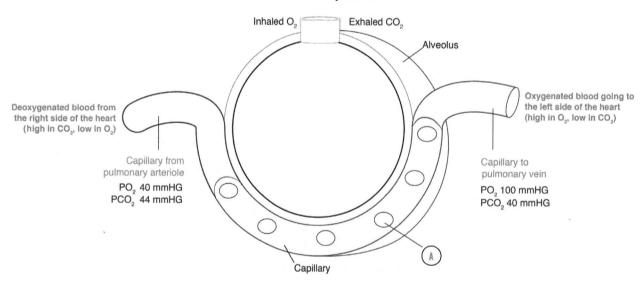

Inhaled O_2 Exhaled CO_2

Alveolus

Deoxygenated blood from the right side of the heart (high in CO_2, low in O_2)

Oxygenated blood going to the left side of the heart (high in O_2, low in CO_2)

Capillary from pulmonary arteriole
PO$_2$ 40 mmHG
PCO$_2$ 44 mmHG

Capillary to pulmonary vein
PO$_2$ 100 mmHG
PCO$_2$ 40 mmHG

Ⓐ

Capillary

External respiration

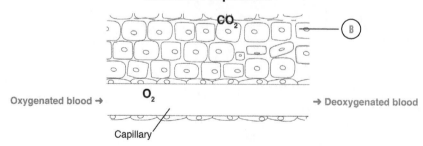

CO$_2$
Ⓑ

Oxygenated blood →
O$_2$
→ Deoxygenated blood

Capillary

CHAPTER 11

THE RENAL SYSTEM: FLUID, ELECTROLYTE AND ACID-BASE BALANCE

INTRODUCTION

Fluid and electrolyte balance and pH (acid–base balance), regulated by the renal system, are essential for normal cell function, particularly in relation to function of nerve and muscle cells. This chapter will help you to revise the structure and functions of the renal system. It will also help you to review your understanding of how fluid moves between compartments in the body. Remember to revise Chapter 11 in *Essentials of Anatomy and Physiology for Nursing Practice*.

Answers to the labelling exercises can be found at the back of the book.

OSMOSIS

INTRODUCTION

Osmosis is the movement of water across a semipermeable membrane from a dilute/hypotonic solution (with low osmotic pressure) to a more concentrated/hypertonic solution (which has a higher osmotic pressure). This works to achieve fluid with similar distribution of water and concentration of solute (substance distributed) in the solvent (water in this case) on both sides of the membrane.

COLOURING NOTES 11.1

☐ Identify the sugar molecules and colour them yellow.

☐ Identify the water molecules and colour them blue.

☐ Label the broken lines.

☐ For the hypertonic solution, using an arrow, identify the direction of movement of the water molecules.

See p. 287 of *Essentials of Anatomy and Physiology for Nursing Practice* to check the answers.

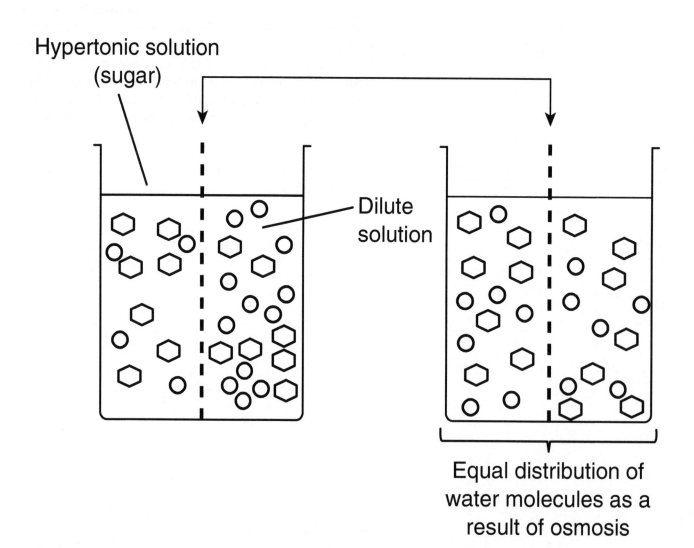

Hypertonic solution (sugar)

Dilute solution

Equal distribution of water molecules as a result of osmosis

EFFECT OF WATER CONCENTRATION ON RED BLOOD CELLS

INTRODUCTION

The tonicity of a fluid refers to the force exerted by osmotically active particles within that fluid. Hypotonic solutions lose water to an isotonic or hypertonic solution in another fluid filled space. Hypertonic solutions gain water from isotonic and hypotonic solutions in another fluid filled space. An example would be the blood as one solution and the fluid within a cell as another solution. The cell membrane separates the two solutions.

COLOURING NOTES 11.2

- ☐ Colour the water blue in each of the three containers.
- ☐ Identify and label the solute. Colour the solutes in all containers green.
- ☐ Identify the erythrocyte in each of the containers. Colour them red.
- ☐ Using arrows, indicate the movement of water between the solution and the erythrocyte in all three containers.

See p. 287 of *Essentials of Anatomy and Physiology for Nursing Practice* to check the answers.

Isotanic solution
(normal)

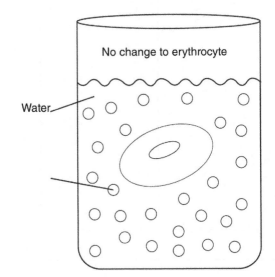

No change to erythrocyte

Water

Hypotonic solution
(dilute)

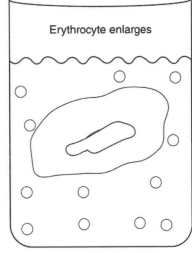

Erythrocyte enlarges

Hypertonic solution
(concentrated)

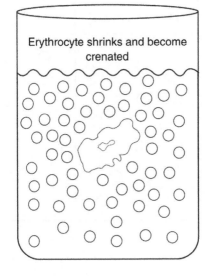

Erythrocyte shrinks and become crenated

DIFFUSION

INTRODUCTION

Diffusion is the movement of ions and molecules from an area of high concentration to an area of low concentration in an attempt to achieve an isotonic balance. It is an important method of achieving a balance of concentration across membranes.

―――――――――――――――――――――――――――― **COLOURING NOTES 11.3** ――――――――――――――

☐ Colour the water blue.
☐ Colour the ions (solute) orange.
☐ Using an arrow, indicate the movement of ions between the compartments to achieve a balanced concentration.

See p. 288 of *Essentials of Anatomy and Physiology for Nursing Practice* to check the answers.

High concentration   Low concentration

Balanced concentration

Equal distribution of
solutes as a result of
diffusion

The Nurse's Anatomy and Physiology Colouring Book published 2017 by SAGE Publishing. © Jennifer Boore, Neal Cook and Andrea Shepherd.

FILTRATION IN THE GLOMERULUS OF THE KIDNEY

INTRODUCTION

In the glomerulus of the kidney, the pressure in the glomerular capillary is greater than in the Bowman's capsule. This forces smaller molecules through the membrane, leaving the cells and larger molecules in the blood. The smaller molecules and fluid that has moved into the Bowman's capsule is called the filtrate.

—— COLOURING NOTES 11.4 ——

☐ Using an arrow, draw the direction of filtrate movement.
☐ Identify and label the afferent and efferent arteriole and the glomerular capillary. Colour them pink.
☐ Colour the blood cells and large molecules red.
☐ Colour the small molecules blue.
☐ Identify and label the Bowman's capsule and tubule. Colour them green.

See p. 289 of *Essentials of Anatomy and Physiology for Nursing Practice* to check the answers.

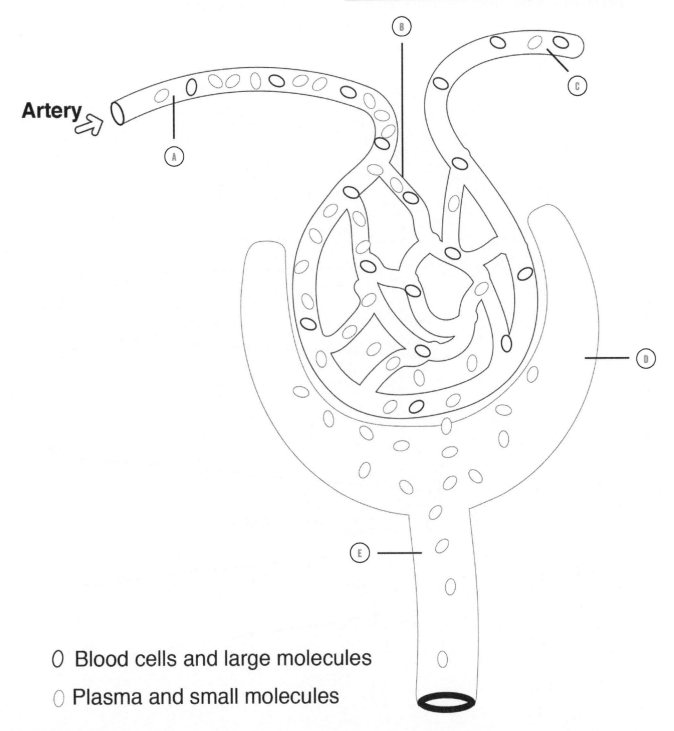

Artery

○ Blood cells and large molecules

○ Plasma and small molecules

THE RENAL SYSTEM

INTRODUCTION

The renal system is one of the excretory systems of the body and is composed of two kidneys, two ureters (one from each kidney) which transport urine to the bladder, and one urethra enabling excretion of urine from the body. The renal system has a number of key functions: excretion (removal of organic wastes from body fluids); elimination (discharge of waste products); and homeostatic regulation.

COLOURING NOTES 11.5

☐ Identify and label the adrenal glands. Colour them green.
☐ Identify and label the kidneys. Colour them red.
☐ Identify and label the ureters. Colour them orange.

☐ Identify and label the bladder. Colour it yellow.
☐ Identify and label the urethra. Colour it blue.
☐ Colour all the bones grey.

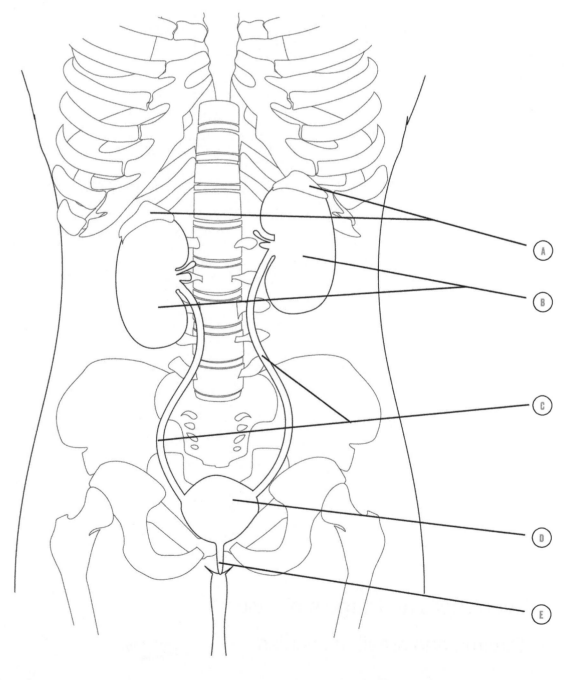

STRUCTURE OF THE KIDNEY

INTRODUCTION

The kidneys are positioned on the posterior wall of the abdomen within the peritoneal cavity. They are about 11–14 cm (4.3–5.5 inches) in length, 6 cm (2.4 inches) wide and 4 cm (1.6 inches) thick. There are two distinct regions within the kidney: the renal cortex and the renal medulla.

─── **COLOURING NOTES 11.6** ───

☐ Identify and label the following:
- ○ Cortex
- ○ Medulla
- ○ Renal lobe
- ○ Renal papilla
- ○ Renal sinus.

☐ Identify and label the minor calyx and major calyx. Colour them blue.

☐ Identify and label the adipose tissue. Colour it yellow.

☐ Identify and label a renal pyramid. Colour them all orange.

☐ Identify and label the renal columns. Colour them green.

☐ Identify and label the renal capsule. Colour it purple.

☐ Identify and label the ureter. Colour it red.

☐ Identify and label the renal pelvis. Colour it pink.

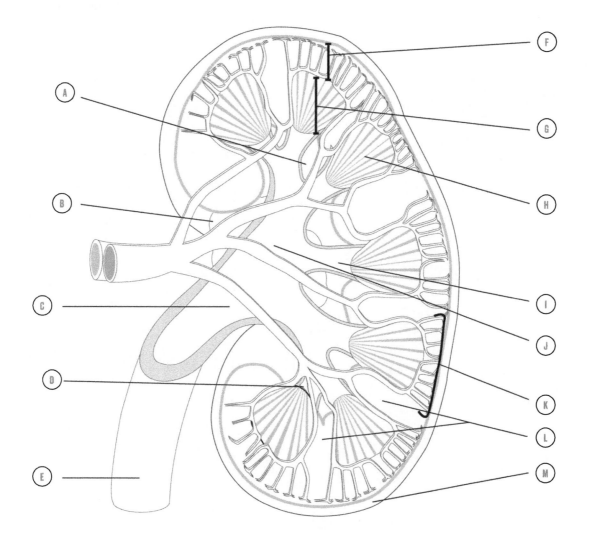

STRUCTURE AND FUNCTION OF THE NEPHRON

INTRODUCTION

Each nephron consists of a renal corpuscle, a spherical structure consisting of the glomerulus and the glomerular (Bowman's) capsule and the renal tubule, which consists of a long tubular passageway divided into the Proximal Convoluted Tubule (PCT), loop of Henle and the Distal Convoluted Tubule (DCT). The nephron undertakes different processes in the formation of urine.

COLOURING NOTES 11.7

- ☐ Identify and label the following:
  - ○ Efferent arteriole
  - ○ Afferent arteriole.

- ☐ Identify and label the Bowman's capsule. Colour it pink.
- ☐ Identify and label the collecting duct. Colour it blue.
- ☐ Identify and label the distal convoluted tubule. Colour it green.
- ☐ Identify and label the glomerulus. Colour it red.

- ☐ Identify and label the loop of Henle, descending limb and ascending limb. Colour them orange.
- ☐ Identify and label the proximal convoluted tubule. Colour it yellow.
- ☐ Using arrows, identify the flow of filtrate through the nephron.

See p. 298 of *Essentials of Anatomy and Physiology for Nursing Practice* to check the answers.

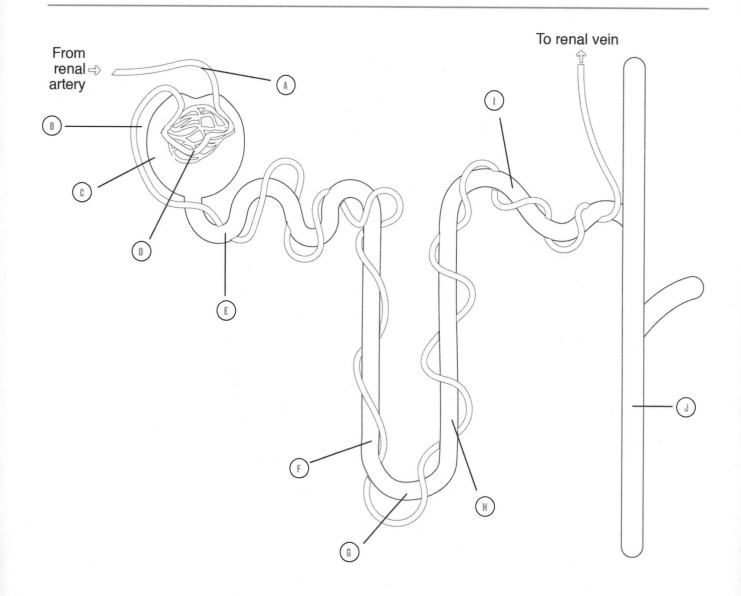

THE BLADDER

INTRODUCTION

The bladder is a muscular, elastic sac that sits on the pelvic floor. It stores urine until it becomes full and urine is eliminated. When empty, the bladder walls fold into ridges or rugae. As the bladder fills these unfold increasing the volume which can be held. The volume held is very variable but 600–800 ml has been reported, with a point of 150–300 ml at which micturition may occur.

COLOURING NOTES 11.8

- ☐ Identify and label the bladder neck.
- ☐ Identify and label the dome of fundus.
- ☐ Identify and label the rugae.
- ☐ Identify and label the ureteral orifices. Colour them black.

- ☐ Identify and label the ureters. Colour them yellow.
- ☐ Identify and label the urethra. Colour it blue.
- ☐ Identify and label the wall of the bladder. Colour it orange.

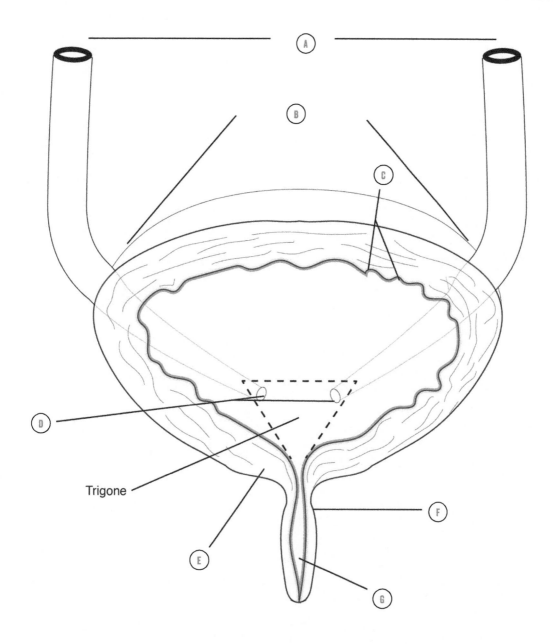

Trigone

CHAPTER 12

THE CARDIOVASCULAR AND LYMPHATIC SYSTEMS: INTERNAL TRANSPORT

INTRODUCTION

Blood and lymph are the key media for transport of substances around the body. The blood and lymphatic vessels are routes for transport of these media. The heart is the pump which provides the force behind the movement of blood and in this chapter will you will revisit the structure and function of the heart. Remember to revise Chapter 12 in *Essentials of Anatomy and Physiology for Nursing Practice*.

Answers to the labelling exercises can be found at the back of the book.

THE HEART AND ITS LOCATION

INTRODUCTION

The heart is effectively two pumps working side by side in one organ, sitting fairly centrally in your chest, with the left lung providing some additional space to the left-hand side. Its location in the thoracic cavity and mediastinum, just behind and to the left of the sternum, means that it is well protected by the sternum and ribcage. It is ideally placed to pump blood against gravity to the brain, and gravity assists the flow to the rest of the body.

--- **COLOURING NOTES 12.1** ---

☐ Identify and label the following:
  ○ Diaphragm
  ○ Oesophagus
  ○ Trachea.
☐ Identify and label the aorta and pulmonary veins. Colour them red.

☐ Identify and label the clavicles. Colour both clavicles yellow.
☐ Identify and label the heart. Colour it pink.
☐ Identify and label the inferior and superior vena cava and pulmonary artery. Colour them blue.
☐ Identify and label the left lung. Colour both lungs purple.

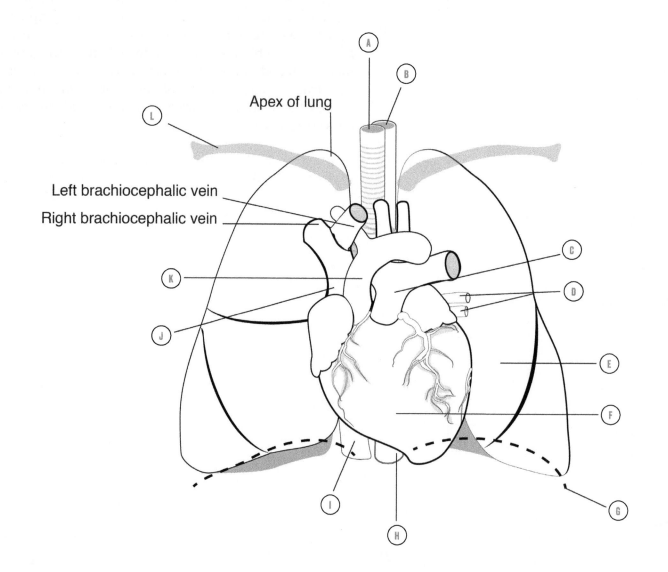

Apex of lung

Left brachiocephalic vein
Right brachiocephalic vein

LAYERS OF THE HEART

INTRODUCTION

The three layers of the heart support its ability to undertake its life-long function as a pump. The pericardium is the outermost layer composed of two sacs which cover the outside of the heart. The middle layer is the myocardium or muscular layer of the heart consisting of thin filaments of actin and thick filaments of myosin. The inner layer is the endocardium which forms the lining of the heart and the heart valves.

COLOURING NOTES 12.2

- ☐ Identify and label the pericardium.
- ☐ Identify and label the endocardium. Colour it purple.
- ☐ Identify and label the fibrous layer. Colour it brown.
- ☐ Identify and label the myocardium. Colour it red.
- ☐ Identify and label the parietal pericardium. Colour it orange.
- ☐ Identify and label the visceral pericardium. Colour it yellow.

The Nurse's Anatomy and Physiology Colouring Book published 2017 by SAGE Publishing. © Jennifer Boore, Neal Cook and Andrea Shepherd.

CIRCULATION AND THE HEART

INTRODUCTION

The heart is comprised of four chambers divided into two sides. Each side of the heart has one atrium and one ventricle, two of each in total. The septum divides the right and left sides of the heart. The role of the atria is to pump blood into the larger ventricles from where it is pumped at force out to its destination.

COLOURING NOTES 12.3

☐ Colour the wall of the heart brown.
☐ Identify and label the aorta and pulmonary veins (left and right). Colour them red.
☐ Identify and label the left atrium and ventricle. Colour them pink.
☐ Identify and label the mitral, tricuspid, pulmonary and aortic valves. Colour them orange.
☐ Identify and label the pulmonary artery and vena cavae (superior and inferior). Colour them dark blue.

☐ Identify and label the right atrium and ventricle. Colour them light blue.
☐ Using black, draw arrows to indicate the direction of blood flow into and out of the heart on both sides.
☐ Using blue, draw arrows to show which blood vessels bring blood from most of the body and out to the lungs.
☐ Using red, draw arrows to show which blood vessels bring blood from the lungs and out to the rest of the body.

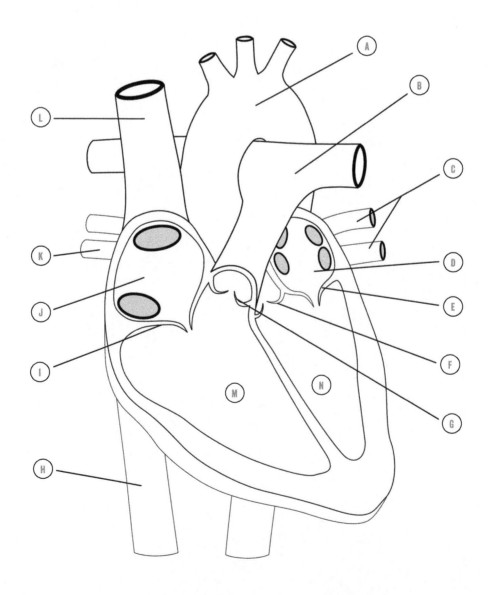

CORONARY CIRCULATION

INTRODUCTION

The coronary circulation supplies blood to the heart itself. Just above the aortic valve lies the opening to the right and left coronary arteries, which supply blood to the heart.

─────── **COLOURING NOTES 12.4** ───────

☐ Identify and label the following:
- ○ Anterior cardiac veins
- ○ Anterior interventricular artery
- ○ Circumflex artery
- ○ Great cardiac vein

- ○ Marginal artery
- ○ Right coronary artery.

☐ Colour all arteries red and veins blue.
☐ Colour the remainder of the heart pink.

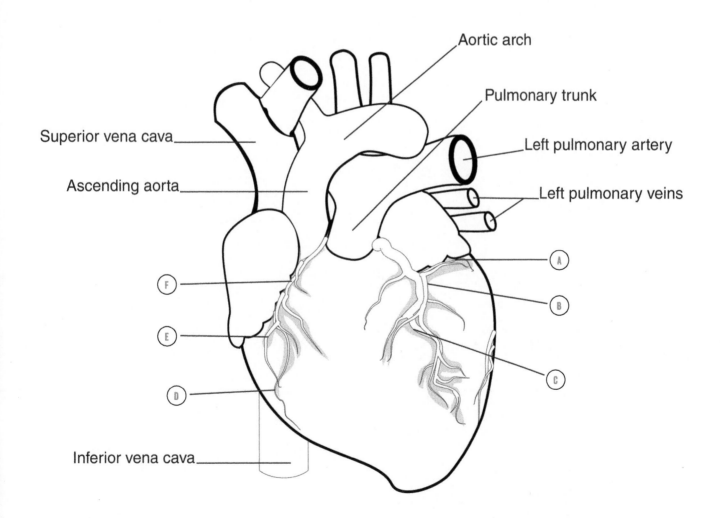

MAJOR ARTERIES OF THE BODY

INTRODUCTION

There are three main types of blood vessels: arteries carry blood away from the heart; capillaries enable exchange of water, nutrients and waste products between the blood and the tissues; and veins carry blood back towards the heart.

COLOURING NOTES 12.5

☐ Identify and label the following, colouring all arteries red:
- ○ Abdominal aorta
- ○ Aorta
- ○ Axillary
- ○ Brachial
- ○ Dorsal pedis
- ○ Femoral
- ○ Internal and external carotid
- ○ Popliteal
- ○ Posterior and anterior tibial
- ○ Radial
- ○ Right and left common carotid
- ○ Ulnar.

☐ Shade the rest of the body in yellow.

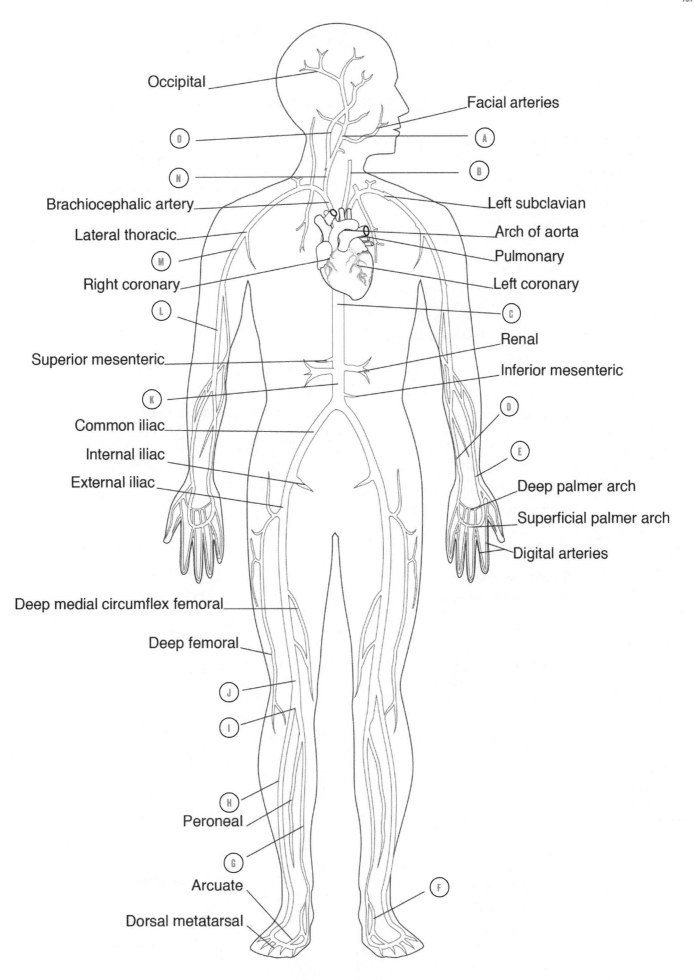

Occipital

Facial arteries

Ⓞ

Ⓐ

Ⓝ

Ⓑ

Brachiocephalic artery

Left subclavian

Lateral thoracic

Arch of aorta

Ⓜ

Pulmonary

Right coronary

Left coronary

Ⓛ

Ⓒ

Renal

Superior mesenteric

Inferior mesenteric

Ⓚ

Ⓓ

Common iliac

Ⓔ

Internal iliac

External iliac

Deep palmer arch

Superficial palmer arch

Digital arteries

Deep medial circumflex femoral

Deep femoral

Ⓙ

Ⓘ

Ⓗ

Peroneal

Ⓖ

Arcuate

Ⓕ

Dorsal metatarsal

The Nurse's Anatomy and Physiology Colouring Book published 2017 by SAGE Publishing. © Jennifer Boore, Neal Cook and Andrea Shepherd.

MAJOR VEINS OF THE BODY

COLOURING NOTES 12.6

☐ Identify and label the following, colouring all veins blue:
- ○ Axillary
- ○ Brachial
- ○ Cephalic
- ○ External and internal jugulars
- ○ Great and small saphenous
- ○ Subclavian.
☐ Shade the rest of the body in yellow.

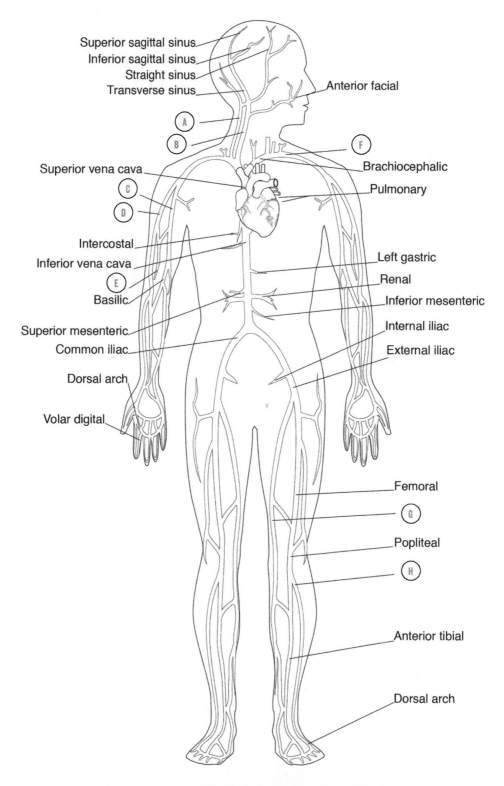

The Nurse's Anatomy and Physiology Colouring Book published 2017 by SAGE Publishing. © Jennifer Boore, Neal Cook and Andrea Shepherd.

STRUCTURE OF BLOOD VESSELS

INTRODUCTION

Arteries and veins have three structural layers similar to all tubular structures:

1. An outer fibrous layer (tunica externa/adventitia).
2. A middle layer of muscle and elastic tissues (tunica media).
3. An inner lining of endothelium which is smooth to facilitate flow of blood (tunica intima).

COLOURING NOTES 12.7

In both images:

☐ Identify and label the lumens. Colour them red.
☐ Identify and label the tunica externa. Colour them green.
☐ Identify and label the tunica intima. Colour them purple.
☐ Identify and label the tunica media. Colour them blue.
☐ Identify and label which of the images is the artery and which is the vein.

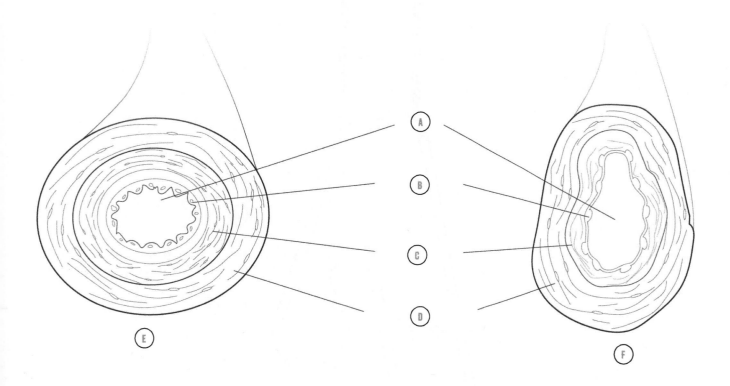

VALVES IN A VEIN

INTRODUCTION

Some veins have valves to prevent the backflow of blood as it is returning towards the heart. Remember, the venous circulation is largely working against gravity in returning blood to the heart and so these valves are necessary.

COLOURING NOTES 12.8

- ☐ Colour the vein blue.
- ☐ Identify and label the valves. Colour them purple.
- ☐ Identify and label the valve cusps.
- ☐ Using black, draw the direction of blood flow on the image.

See p. 328 of *Essentials of Anatomy and Physiology for Nursing Practice* to check the answers.

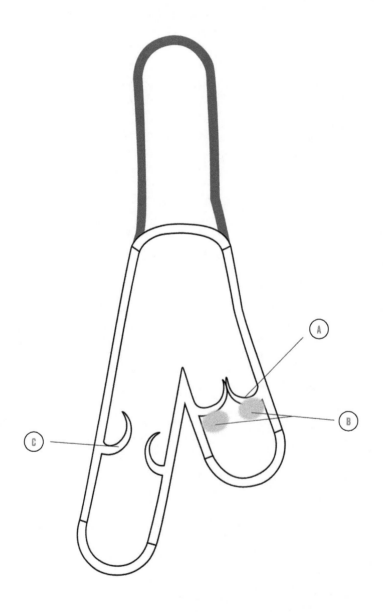

CAPILLARY STRUCTURE

INTRODUCTION

Capillaries are made up of only a single layer of endothelial cells which form a semipermeable membrane that separates the blood and the interstitial fluid compartment

---
COLOURING NOTES 12.9

☐ Identify and label the artery and arteriole. Colour them red.

☐ Identify and label the vein and venule. Colour them blue.

☐ Colour the cells adjacent to the blood vessels yellow. Label them.

☐ Identify and label the capillary wall. Colour the cytoplasm of cells of the capillary wall green and the nuclei black.

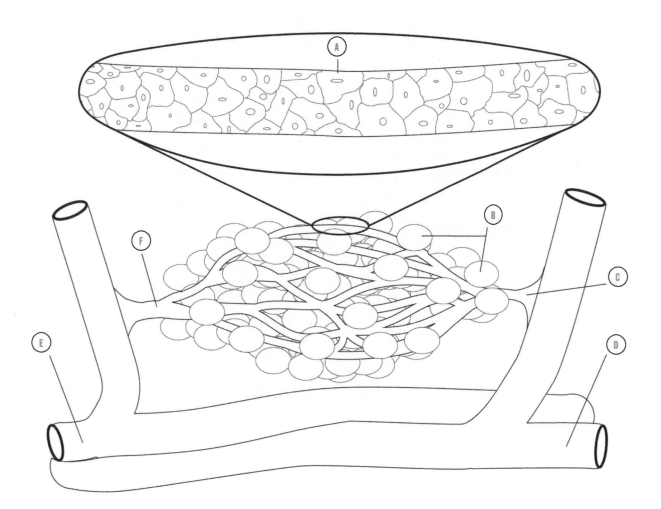

MAJOR LYMPHATIC VESSELS

INTRODUCTION

Lymph flows through the lymphatic vessels and lymph glands that together make up the lymphatic system. Lymphatic vessels have a key role in tissue drainage. The lymphatic system also has a role in the absorption of fat and in immunity.

--- **COLOURING NOTES 12.10** ---

☐ Identify and label the following, colouring all lymphatic vessels green:
- ○ Axillary lymph nodes
- ○ Cervical lymph nodes

- ○ Inguinal lymph nodes
- ○ Left lymphatic duct
- ○ Lumbar lymph nodes
- ○ Popliteal lymph nodes
- ○ Right lymphatic duct

- ○ Thoracic duct
- ○ Thoracic lymph nodes.

☐ Colour the spleen purple.
☐ Colour the heart pink.

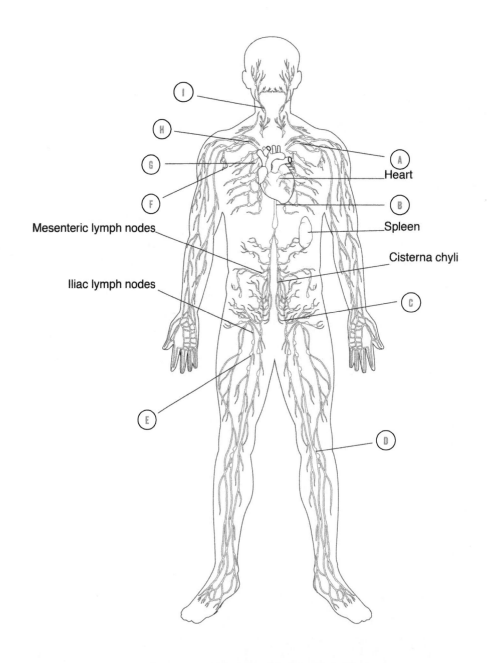

Heart
Spleen
Mesenteric lymph nodes
Cisterna chyli
Iliac lymph nodes

The Nurse's Anatomy and Physiology Colouring Book published 2017 by SAGE Publishing. © Jennifer Boore, Neal Cook and Andrea Shepherd.

LYMPH VESSEL

INTRODUCTION

Lymphatic vessels have a tubular structure similar to that of blood vessels. The lymphatic vessels also have valves to prevent lymph backflow and the smooth muscle in the vessel walls contracts rhythmically to move lymph along. This is assisted by the contraction of adjacent muscles and large arteries.

COLOURING NOTES 12.11

- ☐ Identify and label the valves. Colour them blue.
- ☐ Colour the rest of the vessel green.
- ☐ Colour the lymph yellow.
- ☐ Using black, draw an arrow to show the direction of lymph flow through the vessel.

See p. 331 of *Essentials of Anatomy and Physiology for Nursing Practice* to check the answers.

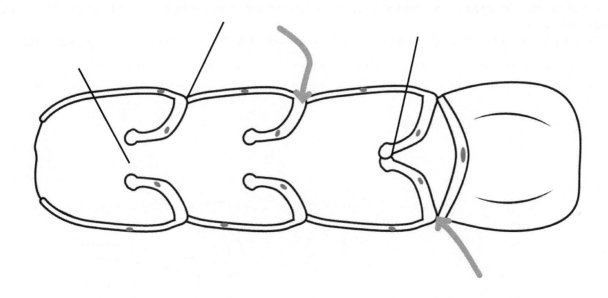

DIFFUSION OF NUTRIENTS AND WASTE PRODUCTS BETWEEN CAPILLARIES AND CELLS

INTRODUCTION

Fluid moves between capillaries and cells primarily as a result of two key forces:

Hydrostatic pressure: This is the pressure exerted by the blood against the artery wall by the force exerted by the heart pumping. This pressure forces fluid and small molecules out of the capillary at the arterial end.

Osmotic pressure: This is the pressure exerted by plasma proteins and some electrolytes in the plasma inside the capillaries. In other words, large plasma proteins, like albumin, and electrolytes, like sodium, pull water towards them. They attract and draw water and small molecules back into the capillary at the venous end.

─────────── **COLOURING NOTES 12.12** ───────────

- ☐ Identify the cells and colour their cytoplasm blue. Colour their nuclei black.
- ☐ Identify and colour the intercellular fluid yellow.
- ☐ Identify and label the lymphatic capillary. Colour it green.
- ☐ Using brown, draw an arrow to indicate the direction and movement of nutrients at the arterial end of the capillary.
- ☐ Using black, draw an arrow to indicate the direction and movement of excess fluid and waste at the venous end of the capillary.
- ☐ Using purple, draw an arrow to indicate the direction of blood flow within the capillary. Colour the blood red.

See p. 333 of *Essentials of Anatomy and Physiology for Nursing Practice* to check the answers.

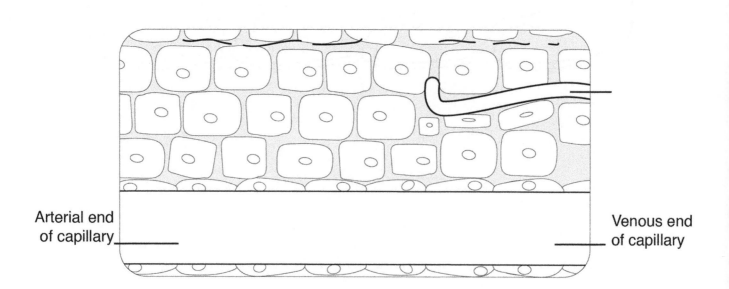

Arterial end of capillary

Venous end of capillary

CONDUCTION SYSTEM OF THE HEART

INTRODUCTION

The conduction system initiates and carries an electrical impulse (nervous impulse through action potentials) across the myocardium, triggering the muscles to contract as it passes.

COLOURING NOTES 12.13

- ☐ Identify and label the right and left atria. Colour them yellow. Colour the corresponding part of the PQRST complex that represents electrical activity in this area yellow.
- ☐ Identify and label the right and left ventricles. Colour them green. Colour the corresponding part of the PQRST complex that represents electrical activity in this area green.
- ☐ Identify and label the atrioventricular node. Colour it blue. Colour the corresponding part of the PQRST complex that represents electrical activity in this area blue.
- ☐ Colour the T wave black.
- ☐ Identify and label the sinoatrial node. Colour it orange.
- ☐ Colour the wall of the heart red.
- ☐ Identify and label the atrioventricular bundle and the bundle branches. Colour them purple.
- ☐ Identify and label the Purkinje fibres.
- ☐ Using black, draw arrows to show the direction of electrical impulses in the cardiac cycle.

See p. 334 of *Essentials of Anatomy and Physiology for Nursing Practice* to check the answers.

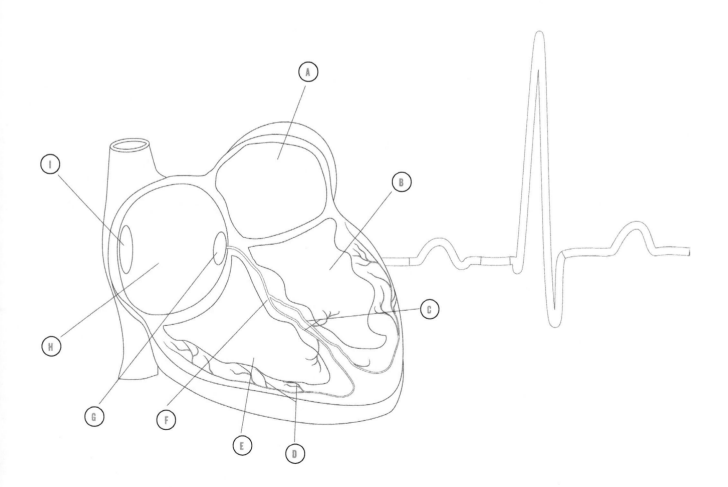

CHAPTER 13

THE IMMUNE SYSTEM: INTERNAL PROTECTION

INTRODUCTION

The immune system plays a crucial role in maintaining health through combating infections and abnormal cells and is important at all stages of life. The immune system consists of two major sections: the innate and adaptive systems, which together provide a considerable degree of protection against infection. The chapter will help you to review the structure and function of the immune system in maintaining health. Remember to revise Chapter 13 in *Essentials of Anatomy and Physiology for Nursing Practice*.

Answers to the labelling exercises can be found at the back of the book.

PHYSICAL AND BIOCHEMICAL BARRIERS TO INFECTION

INTRODUCTION

Physical barriers play an important role in minimising the entry of pathogens into the body. In addition, a number of biochemical substances are formed which protect against pathogens, and the commensal microbes within the microbiome already inhabit sites in the body and prevent pathogens colonising those sites.

COLOURING NOTES 13.1

☐ Identify the bronchi. Write a description of how they contribute to physical and/or biochemical barriers to pathogens. Colour their location blue.

☐ Identify the eyes. Write a description of how they contribute to physical and/or biochemical barriers to pathogens. Colour them grey.

☐ Identify the large intestine. Write a description of how it contributes to physical and/or biochemical barriers to pathogens. Colour it purple.

☐ Identify the nasal cavity. Write a description of how it contributes to physical and/or biochemical barriers to pathogens. Colour it green.

☐ Identify the pharynx. Write a description of how it contributes to physical and/or biochemical barriers to pathogens. Colour it red.

☐ Identify the skin. Write a description of how it contributes to physical and/or biochemical barriers to pathogens. Shade the skin pink.

☐ Identify the small intestine. Write a description of how the lower ileum contributes to physical and/or biochemical barriers to pathogens. Colour the small intestine brown.

☐ Identify the stomach. Write a description of how it contributes to physical and/or biochemical barriers to pathogens. Colour it orange.

☐ Identify the vagina. Write a description of how it contributes to physical and/or biochemical barriers to pathogens. Colour it yellow.

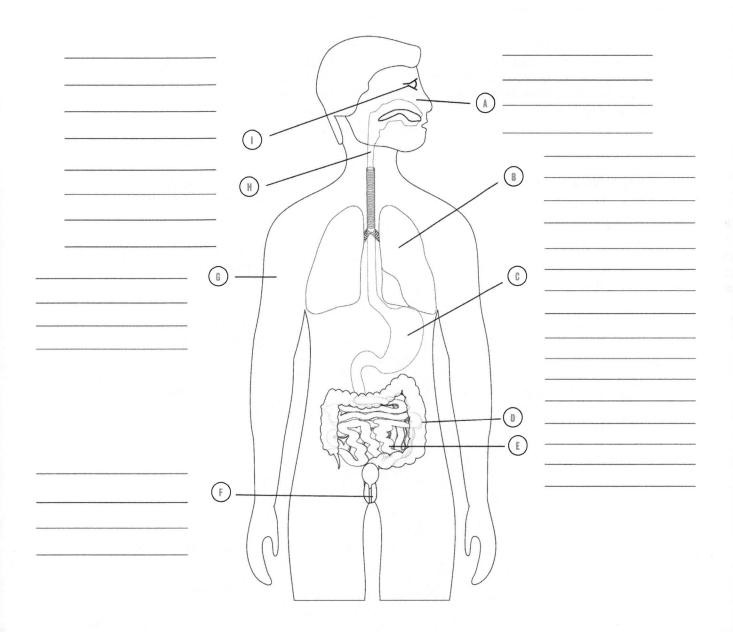

LYMPHOID ORGANS AND TISSUES

INTRODUCTION

The thymus and bone marrow are the two organs involved in formation of the cells of the immune system. There are numerous other organs and tissues where cells of the immune system are located.

COLOURING NOTES 13.2

- ☐ Colour all lymph nodes black.
- ☐ Identify and label the thymus. Colour it green.
- ☐ Identify and label the spleen. Colour it purple.
- ☐ Identify and label the bone marrow. Colour it orange.
- ☐ Colour the lungs blue.

- ☐ Colour the large intestine brown.
- ☐ Colour the small intestine pink.
- ☐ Colour the stomach and oesophagus yellow.
- ☐ Colour the liver red.
- ☐ Colour the pancreas grey.

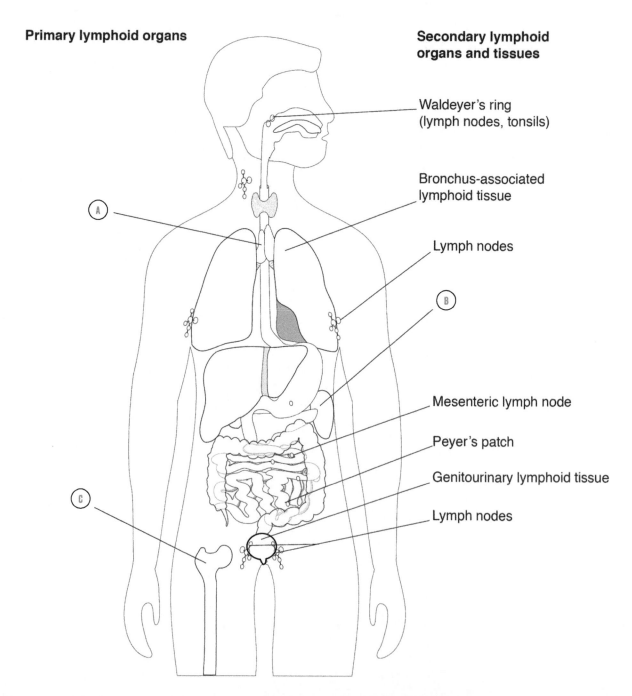

Primary lymphoid organs

Secondary lymphoid organs and tissues

Waldeyer's ring
(lymph nodes, tonsils)

Bronchus-associated
lymphoid tissue

Lymph nodes

A

B

Mesenteric lymph node

Peyer's patch

Genitourinary lymphoid tissue

Lymph nodes

C

IMMUNITY

INTRODUCTION

Immunity is the state when an individual has resistance to infection or disease, developed through the innate and/or adaptive immune mechanisms. It can be natural or artificial in development and active or passive in nature

---
COLOURING NOTES 13.3

- ☐ Fill in the missing words in the diagram below.
- ☐ Colour the passive immunity sections green
- ☐ Colour the active immunity sections pink.

See p. 363 of *Essentials of Anatomy and Physiology for Nursing Practice* to check the answers.

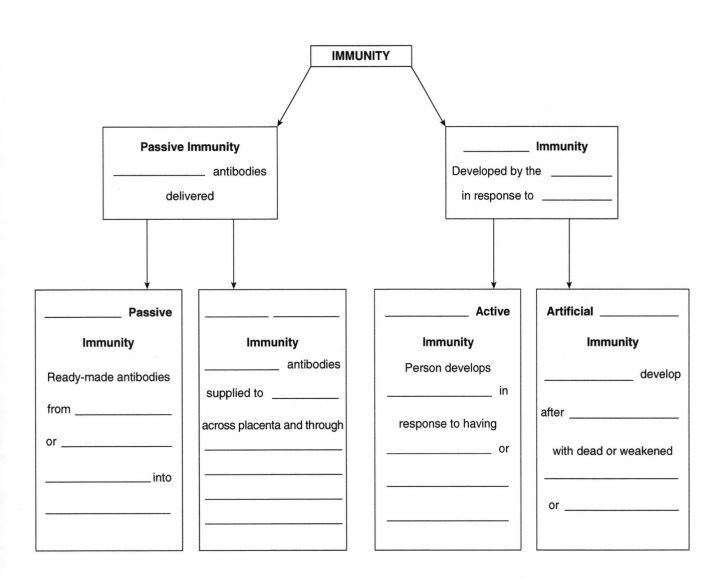

CHAPTER 14

SKIN AND TEMPERATURE REGULATION

INTRODUCTION

The skin protects the body in numerous ways, contributing to homeostasis. Human cells function optimally at a specific body temperature, and the skin plays a major role in temperature regulation. This chapter will help you to review the anatomical and physiological knowledge necessary to underpin the functions of skin and thermoregulation. Remember to revise Chapter 14 in *Essentials of Anatomy and Physiology for Nursing Practice*.

Answers to the labelling exercises can be found at the back of the book.

LAYERS OF THE SKIN

INTRODUCTION

The skin is the largest organ in the body and has an approximate surface area of 1.8–2 m². It is a multifunctional organ that plays a pivotal role in maintaining homeostasis through various functions. The skin has numerous accessory structures, largely within the dermis.

COLOURING NOTES 14.1

☐ Identify and label the following:
- ○ Dermis
- ○ Epidermis
- ○ Hypodermis
- ○ Papillary layer
- ○ Reticular layer
- ○ Sweat pore.

☐ Colour the epidermis light blue.

☐ Identify and label the arrector pili muscle. Colour it orange.

☐ Colour the artery red.

☐ Colour the fat cells yellow.

☐ Identify and label a hair shaft and follicle. Colour the hair shafts and follicles black.

☐ Identify and label the lamellated corpuscle. Colour it navy.

☐ Identify and label a nerve fibre. Colour it pink.

☐ Identify and label the sebaceous gland. Colour it yellow.

☐ Identify and label the sweat gland and duct. Colour them brown.

☐ Identify and label the tactile corpuscle. Colour it green.

☐ Colour the vein blue.

See p. 376 of *Essentials of Anatomy and Physiology for Nursing Practice* to check the answers.

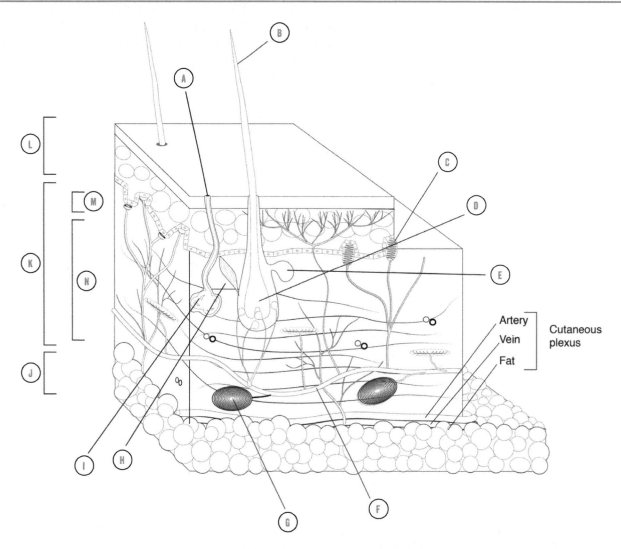

STAGES OF WOUND HEALING

INTRODUCTION

Whether a wound heals by primary, secondary or tertiary intention, it will go through a number of stages of healing. Different sources refer to differing numbers of stages of healing, but most agree that there are four key stages. They are:

1. Haemostasis.
2. Inflammation.
3. Proliferation (migration, granulation and proliferation).
4. Maturation (and remodelling).

--- **COLOURING NOTES 14.2** ---

HAEMOSTASIS AND INFLAMMATION

- ☐ Identify and label the capillary. Colour it red.
- ☐ Identify and label the epithelial cells. Colour them light blue.
- ☐ Identify and label the fibroblasts. Colour these green.
- ☐ Identify and label the neutrophils. Colour them orange.

- ☐ Identify and label the platelets. Colour them purple.
- ☐ Colour the epidermis dark blue.
- ☐ Colour the dermis pink.
- ☐ Colour the subcutaneous layer yellow.

Haemostasis and Inflammation

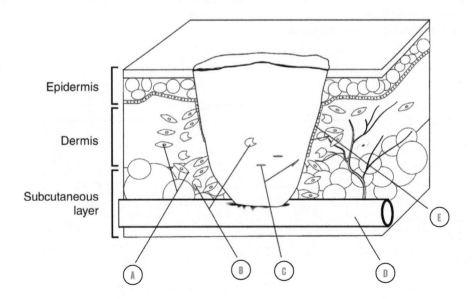

Epidermis

Dermis

Subcutaneous layer

PROLIFERATION

- ☐ Identify and label the eschar. Colour it black.
- ☐ Identify and label the new blood vessel.
- ☐ Identify and label the granulation tissue. Colour it red.
- ☐ Colour the epidermis blue.
- ☐ Colour the dermis pink.
- ☐ Colour the subcutaneous layer yellow.
- ☐ Identify and label the fibroblasts. Colour these green.
- ☐ Identify and label the neutrophils. Colour them orange.

Proliferation

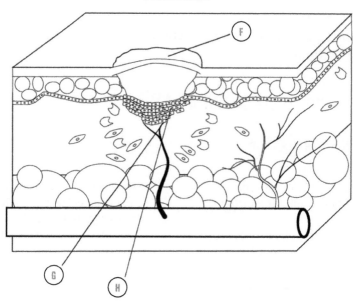

MATURATION

- ☐ Colour the epidermis blue.
- ☐ Colour the dermis pink.
- ☐ Colour the subcutaneous layer yellow.
- ☐ Colour the scar tissue red and the surrounding skin light brown

- ☐ Identify and label the fibroblasts. Colour these green.
- ☐ Identify and label the neutrophils. Colour them orange.

Maturation

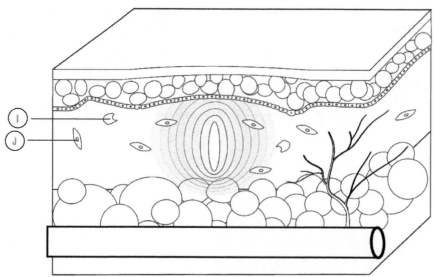

MECHANISM OF HEAT LOSS

INTRODUCTION

There are four key mechanisms for heat loss from the body:

- Radiation.
- Conduction.
- Convection.
- Evaporation.

COLOURING NOTES 14.3

☐ Beside each mechanism of heat loss, write a small description of how this type of heat loss occurs.
☐ Shade the body in red.

See p. 391 of *Essentials of Anatomy and Physiology for Nursing Practice* to check the answers.

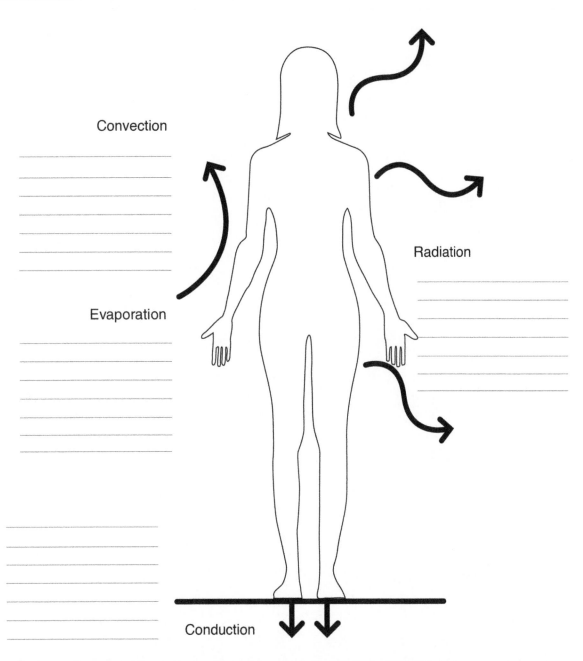

Convection

Radiation

Evaporation

Conduction

THERMOREGULATION

INTRODUCTION

The hypothalamus is the control centre with information on body temperature received and actions initiated to adjust the balance between heat production and heat loss to maintain the correct body temperature.

―――――――――――――――― **COLOURING NOTES 14.4** ――――――――――――――――

☐ Fill in the missing words in the diagram.
☐ Colour the sections of the negative feedback mechanism orange.
☐ Colour the cooling mechanisms section blue.
☐ Colour the warming mechanisms green.
☐ Colour both stimuli sections yellow.
☐ Colour the arrows black.

See p. 390 of *Essentials of Anatomy and Physiology for Nursing Practice* to check the answers.

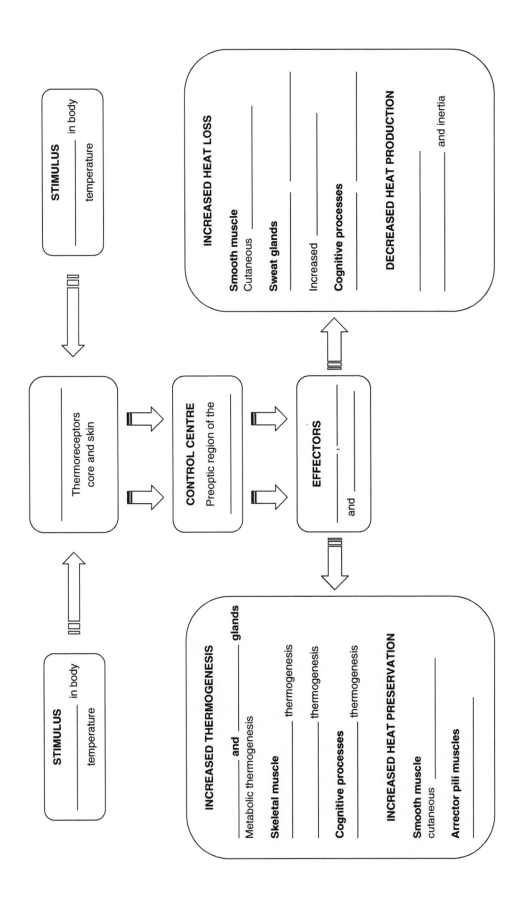

STIMULUS
_____ in body
temperature

Thermoreceptors
_____
core and skin

CONTROL CENTRE
Preoptic region of the
_____

EFFECTORS
_____
and _____

INCREASED HEAT LOSS

Smooth muscle
Cutaneous _____

Sweat glands
Increased _____

Cognitive processes
_____

DECREASED HEAT PRODUCTION
_____ and inertia

STIMULUS
_____ in body
temperature

INCREASED THERMOGENESIS
_____ and
_____ glands
Metabolic thermogenesis

Skeletal muscle
_____ thermogenesis
_____ thermogenesis

Cognitive processes
_____ thermogenesis

INCREASED HEAT PRESERVATION

Smooth muscle
cutaneous _____

Arrector pili muscles
_____

CHAPTER 15

THE MUSCULOSKELETAL SYSTEM: SUPPORT AND MOVEMENT

INTRODUCTION

The musculoskeletal system is vital to how we function physically; it provides the framework for your body, creates movements, permits flexibility and provides protection for various organs. This chapter will help you to review the structure of the musculoskeletal (i.e. skeleton and muscles) system. Remember to revise Chapter 15 in *Essentials of Anatomy and Physiology for Nursing Practice*.

Answers to the labelling exercises can be found at the back of the book.

THE SKELETON

INTRODUCTION

The adult human skeleton contains 206 bones. A child's skeleton is mostly cartilage that through the process of ossification eventually becomes bone. A child has considerably more bones (300–350) many of which fuse together to form the 206 bones of the adult skeleton.

The human skeleton is divided into two parts: the axial skeleton and the appendicular skeleton.

COLOURING NOTES 15.1

- ☐ Label the identified bones.
- ☐ Colour the axial skeleton blue.
- ☐ Colour the appendicular skeleton orange.

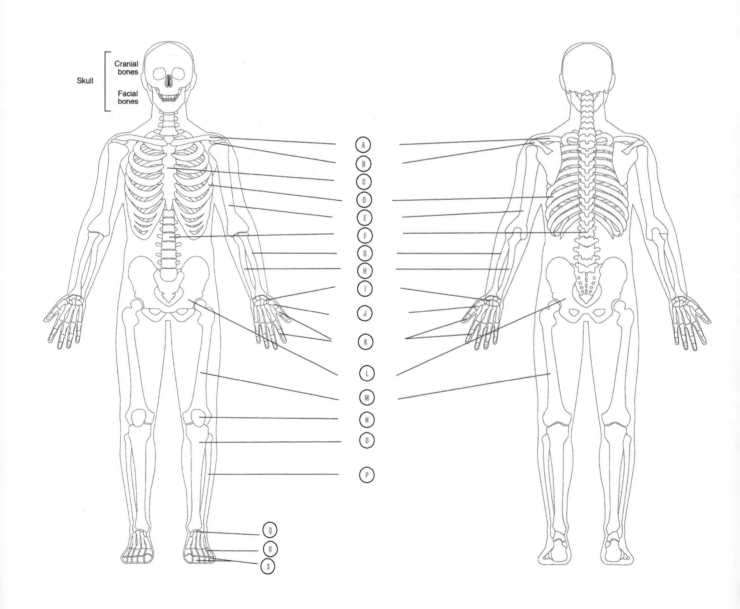

STRUCTURE OF A LONG BONE

INTRODUCTION

The structure of a bone can be discussed in terms of the parts of a long bone. This is one that is longer in length than width, e.g. the femur (thigh bone). A long bone consists of the following parts: diaphysis, epiphysis, metaphysis, articular cartilage, periosteum, medullary cavity and endosteum.

─── COLOURING NOTES 15.2 ───

- ☐ Identify and label the:
  - ○ Epiphysis
  - ○ Diaphysis
  - ○ Nutrient foramen
  - ○ Epiphyseal line.
- ☐ Identify and label the blood vessel. Colour it red.

- ☐ Identify and label the articular cartilage. Colour it grey.
- ☐ Identify and label the compact bone. Colour it purple.
- ☐ Identify and label the endosteum. Colour it yellow.
- ☐ Identify and label the medullary cavity. Colour it pink.
- ☐ Identify and label the periosteum. Colour it orange.
- ☐ Identify and label the spongy bone. Colour it green.

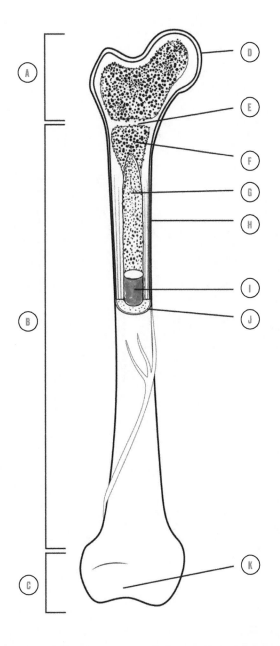

COMPACT BONE

INTRODUCTION

This is the strongest type of bone tissue. It is dense and contains few spaces, thus offering a high degree of protection and support for the bone to withstand the pressures exerted by weight and movement. This type of bone is found beneath the periosteum of all bones and accounts for the majority of the diaphyses of long bones.

COLOURING NOTES 15.3

- ☐ Identify and label the blood vessels within the central canal and perforating canal. Colour them red and blue.
- ☐ Identify and label the circumferential, concentric and interstitial lamella. Colour all of them orange.
- ☐ Identify and label the osteocytes. Colour them pink.
- ☐ Identify and label the osteon.
- ☐ Identify and label the periosteum. Colour it grey.

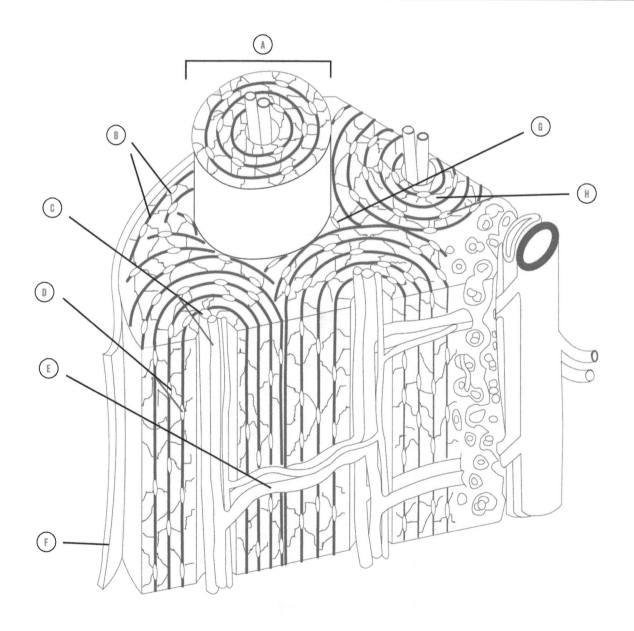

SPONGY BONE

INTRODUCTION

Spongy bone is always found inside the bone and is protected by a layer of compact bone. It tends to be found in bones that have low levels of stress or where pressures are exerted from a range of directions. The spaces mean that spongy bone is much lighter than compact bone thereby reducing the overall weight of bones, allowing them to move easily when pulled by skeletal muscle.

COLOURING NOTES 15.4

- ☐ Identify and label the spaces containing blood vessels and bone marrow.
- ☐ Identify and label the trabeculae. Colour them pink.
- ☐ Identify the articular cartilage and colour it grey.
- ☐ Identify the blood vessel and colour it red.
- ☐ Identify the compact bone and colour it yellow.

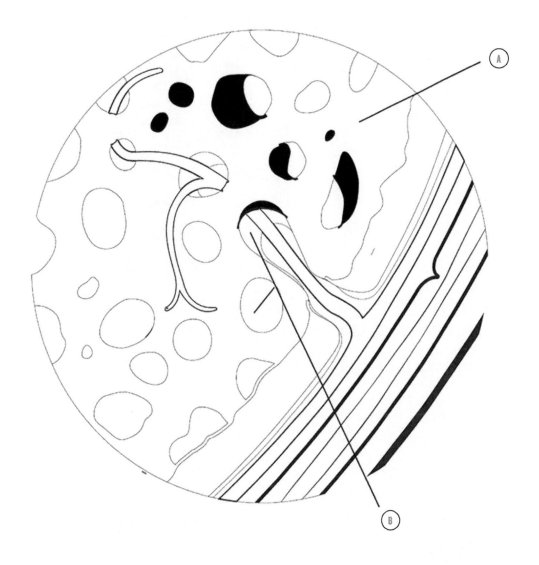

TYPES OF BONE BASED ON SHAPE

INTRODUCTION

Bones can be classified into six types according to their shape: long, short, flat, irregular, sesamoid and sutural.

COLOURING NOTES 15.5

☐ Identify and label a flat bone. Colour it orange.
☐ Identify and label a long bone. Colour it red.
☐ Identify and label a sesamoid bone. Colour it green.

☐ Identify and label a short bone. Colour it purple.
☐ Identify and label a sutural bone. Colour it yellow.
☐ Identify and label an irregular bone. Colour it blue.

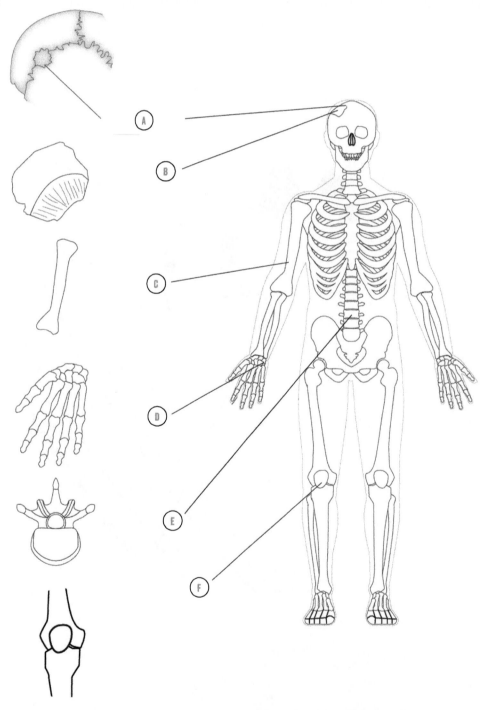

THE CRANIAL BONES

INTRODUCTION

These eight bones form the cranial cavity which encloses and protects the delicate tissue of the brain. The eight cranial bones are: the frontal bone, two parietal bones, two temporal bones, the occipital bone, the sphenoid bone and the ethmoid bone.

COLOURING NOTES 15.6

☐ Identify and label the ethmoid bone. Colour it brown.
☐ Identify and label the frontal bone. Colour it green.
☐ Identify and label the occipital bone. Colour it yellow.
☐ Identify and label the parietal bone. Colour it purple.

☐ Identify and label the sphenoid bone. Colour it blue.
☐ Identify and label the temporal bone. Colour it orange.
☐ Identify and label the mandible. Colour it grey.

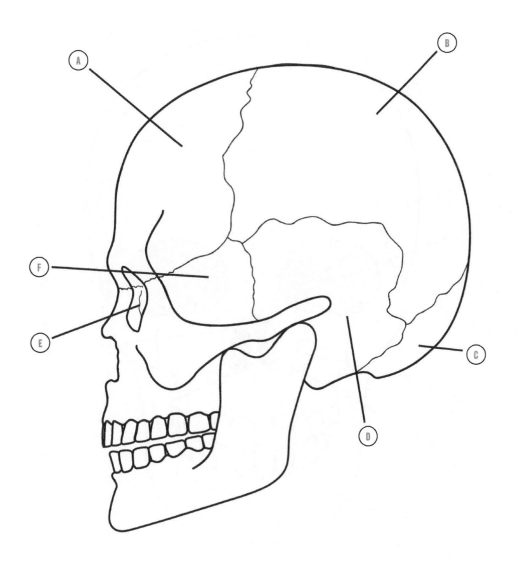

THE FACIAL BONES

INTRODUCTION

Fourteen bones form the face and include: two nasal bones, two maxillae (joined to form the upper jaw), two zygomatic bones (cheekbones), the mandible (jawbone), two lacrimal bones, two palatine bones, two inferior nasal conchae and the vomer.

COLOURING NOTES 15.7

☐ Identify and label the frontal bone.
☐ Identify and label the inferior nasal conchae. Colour them blue.
☐ Identify and label the lacrimal bones and palatine bones.
☐ Identify and label the mandible. Colour it grey.
☐ Identify and label the maxillae. Colour them brown.

☐ Identify and label the nasal bones. Colour them purple.
☐ Identify and label the perpendicular plate of the ethmoid. Colour it yellow.
☐ Identify and label the zygomatic bones. Colour them pink.
☐ Identify and label the vomer. Colour it orange.

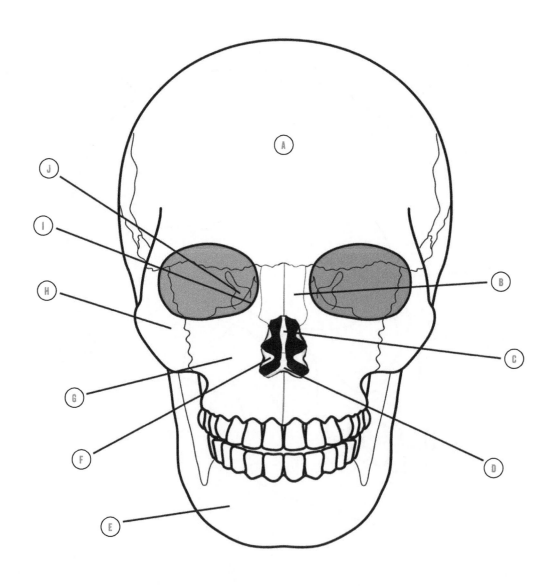

PARTS OF A VERTEBRA

INTRODUCTION

The spinal column consists of 33 vertebrae, the individual bones of the spine that stack up to complete its bony structure. The vertebrae all have a similar shape but the distinct sections have structural modifications necessary for movement and protection. Each vertebra is numbered and the number is preceded by a letter that indicates its section, e.g. C1 is the first vertebra in the cervical spine.

COLOURING NOTES 15.8

- ☐ Identify and label the pedicles. Colour them green.
- ☐ Identify and label the space for the spinal cord.
- ☐ Identify and label the spinous and transverse processes. Colour them blue.
- ☐ Identify and label the vertebral body. Colour it grey.

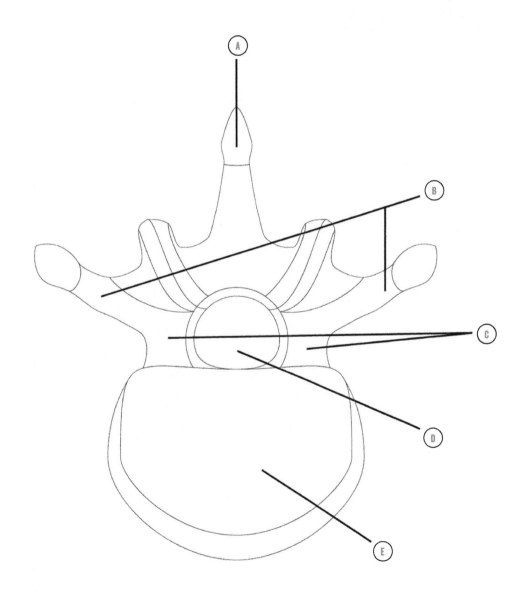

SECTIONS OF THE SPINAL COLUMN

INTRODUCTION

The five sections of spinal vertebrae are (not in this order!):

- Cervical.
- Coccygeal (fused).
- Lumbar.
- Sacral (fused).
- Thoracic.

——— COLOURING NOTES 15.9 ———

☐ Identify and colour the cervical vertebrae orange.
☐ Identify and colour the coccygeal vertebrae grey.
☐ Identify and colour the lumbar vertebrae yellow.
☐ Identify and colour the sacral vertebrae blue.
☐ Identify and colour the thoracic vertebrae green.

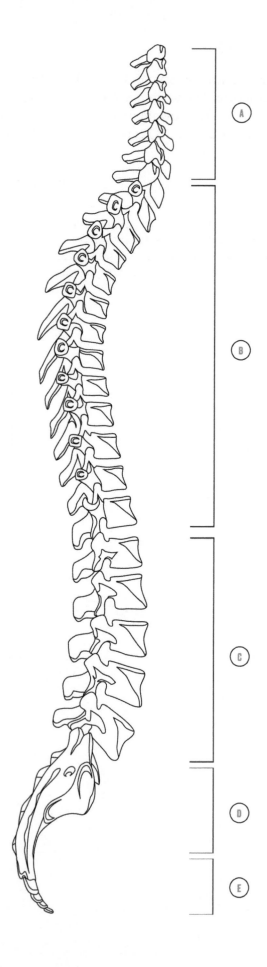

BONES OF THE THORAX

INTRODUCTION

Bones of the thorax protect the organs contained within the thoracic cavity, e.g. the heart and lungs. They include the sternum (breast bone) and ribs.

—————— **COLOURING NOTES 15.10** ——————

☐ Identify and label:
- ○ Clavicular notch
- ○ Costal cartilage
- ○ False ribs
- ○ Floating ribs
- ○ Manubrium
- ○ Sternal angle

- ○ Sternal body
- ○ Sternum
- ○ True ribs
- ○ Xiphoid process.

☐ Colour the sternum green.
☐ Colour the ribs blue.

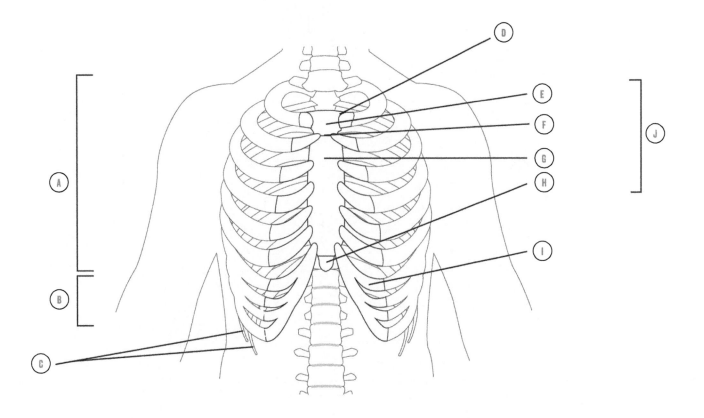

BONES OF THE PECTORAL GIRDLE AND UPPER EXTREMITIES

INTRODUCTION

The pectoral girdle attaches the bones of the upper limbs to the axial skeleton and consists of a clavicle and a scapula on each side. There are 30 bones in each of the upper limbs: humerus, ulna and radius (forearm), eight carpal bones in the wrist, five metacarpals in the palm and 14 phalanges (bones in the digits).

—— COLOURING NOTES 15.11 ——

- ☐ Identify and label the carpals. Colour them red.
- ☐ Identify and label the clavicle. Colour it yellow.
- ☐ Identify and label the humerus. Colour it blue.
- ☐ Identify and label the metacarpals. Colour them pink.
- ☐ Identify and label the phalanges. Colour them purple.

- ☐ Identify and label the radius. Colour it green.
- ☐ Identify and label the scapula. Colour it orange.
- ☐ Identify and label the ulna. Colour it brown.
- ☐ Label the pectoral girdle.

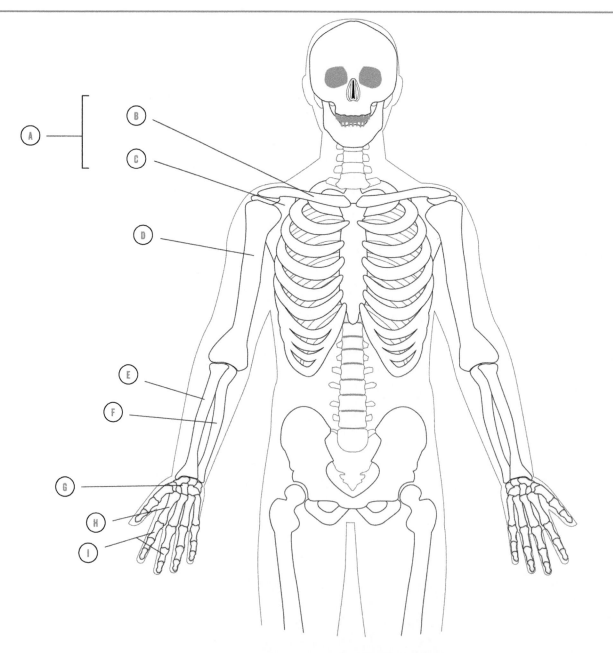

THE PELVIC GIRDLE

INTRODUCTION

The pelvic girdle is made up of two pelvic bones (hip bones). In adults each hip bone is made up of three components: ilium, ischium and pubis. In infants and children these are not fused and are separated by cartilage. As a child matures into adulthood, they fuse to form the adult hip bone by around the age of 23. The hip bones join at the front (anterior) at the pubic symphysis and at the back (posterior) with the sacrum; together they form the bony pelvis

—————————————— COLOURING NOTES 15.12 ——————————————

☐ Identify and label an acetabulum. Colour both blue.
☐ Identify and label the coccyx. Colour it pink.
☐ Identify and label an ileum. Colour both purple.
☐ Identify and label the iliac crest.
☐ Identify and label an ischium. Colour both green.

☐ Identify and label the pubic bone. Colour it grey.
☐ Identify and label the pubic crest.
☐ Identify and label the sacrum. Colour it yellow.
☐ Identify and label the symphysis. Colour it orange.

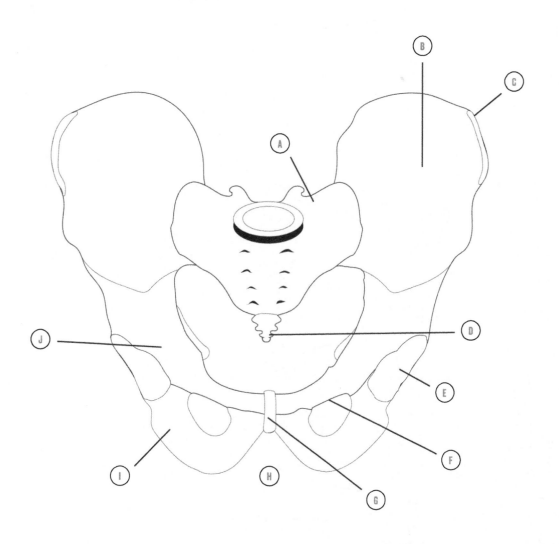

BONES OF THE LOWER EXTREMITIES

INTRODUCTION

The lower extremities consist of 30 bones: femur, patella (kneecap), tibia and fibula, seven tarsal bones (ankle), five metatarsals and 14 phalanges (bones of the digits).

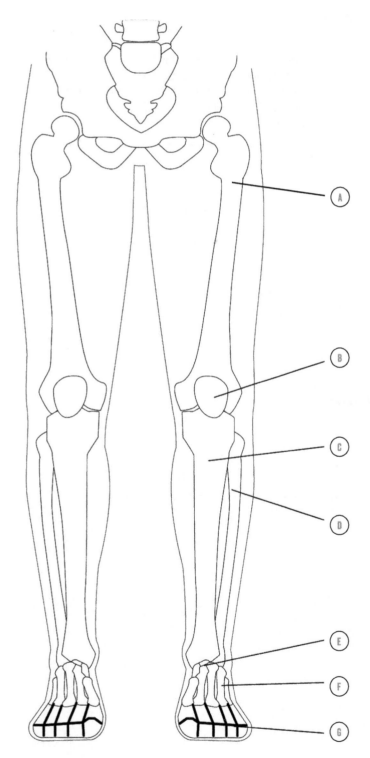

─── COLOURING NOTES 15.13 ───

- ☐ Identify and label a femur. Colour both blue.
- ☐ Identify and label a patella. Colour both green.
- ☐ Identify and label a tibia. Colour both yellow.
- ☐ Identify and label a fibula. Colour both red.
- ☐ Identify and label the tarsals. Colour them purple.
- ☐ Identify and label the metatarsals. Colour them pink.
- ☐ Identify and label the phalanges. Colour them orange.

SYNOVIAL JOINT

INTRODUCTION

This type of joint is the most common type in the body. A synovial joint has a distinct characteristic in having a space, the synovial cavity, between the ends of the articulating bones. The large range of movement in synovial joints defines them functionally as diarthroses as they are freely movable. Friction at the articulating surfaces is low because the articular cartilage is elastic and the joint is filled with fluid. Synovial joints all have the same characteristics and contain an articular cartilage, an articular capsule and a joint cavity.

COLOURING NOTES 15.14

- ☐ Identify and label the articular capsule. Colour it blue.
- ☐ Identify and label the articular cartilage. Colour it grey.
- ☐ Identify and label the bone. Colour it yellow.
- ☐ Identify and label the synovial fluid. Colour it green.
- ☐ Identify and label the synovial membrane. Colour it orange.

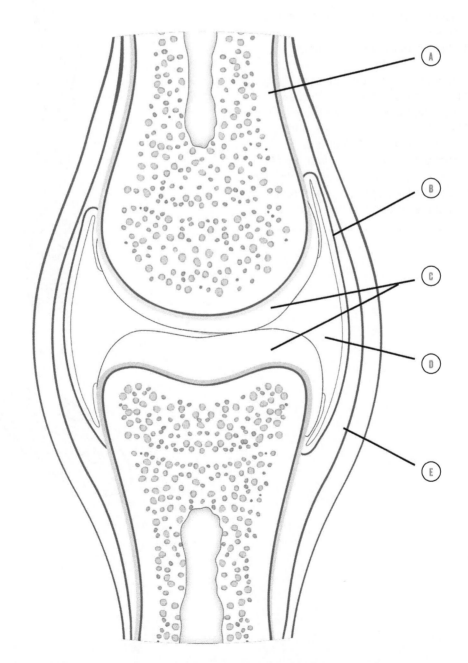

COMPONENTS OF SKELETAL MUSCLE

INTRODUCTION

Skeletal muscle is the most abundant of the three types of muscle in the body accounting for approximately 40–50% of a person's total body weight. Skeletal muscle is striated (when looked at under a microscope it appears to have light and dark stripes) and is under voluntary control of the nervous system. It has four key functions: production of body movements, maintaining body position, storage and movement, and generation of heat.

—— COLOURING NOTES 15.15 ——

☐ Identify and label the actin and myosin filaments. Colour them blue.
☐ Identify and label the blood vessels. Colour them red.
☐ Identify and label the epimysium. Colour it orange.
☐ Identify and label the fascicle. Colour it yellow.
☐ Identify and label the fasciculi. Colour them green.
☐ Identify and label the myofibril. Shade it purple.
☐ Identify and label the nucleus. Colour it black.
☐ Identify and label the perimysium. Colour it pink.
☐ Identify and label the sarcolemma and endomysium.
☐ Identify and label the sarcomere. Colour it red.
☐ Identify and label the striations.

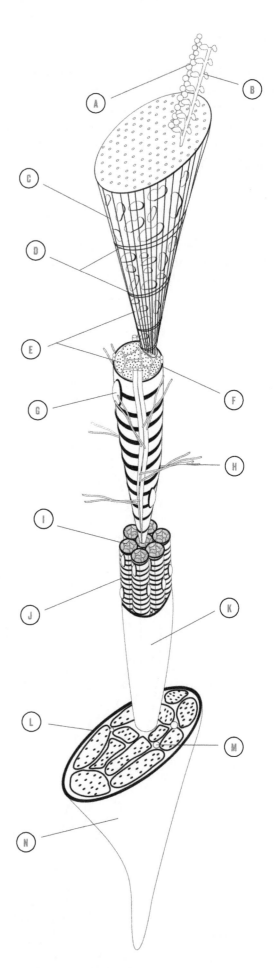

MUSCULATURE OF THE BODY

INTRODUCTION

Muscles can be named according to several factors: shape, size, location and number of insertions. The skeletal muscles can be grouped into four areas:

1. Head and neck.
2. Upper limbs.
3. Thorax and abdomen.
4. Lower limbs.

MUSCLES OF THE HEAD AND NECK

COLOURING NOTES 15.16

- ☐ Identify and label the orbicularis oculi muscle. Colour it blue.
- ☐ Identify and label the orbicularis oris muscle. Colour it red.
- ☐ Identify and label the sternocleidomastoid muscle. Colour it green.
- ☐ Identify and label the trapezius muscle. Colour it yellow.
- ☐ Colour the remaining muscles orange.

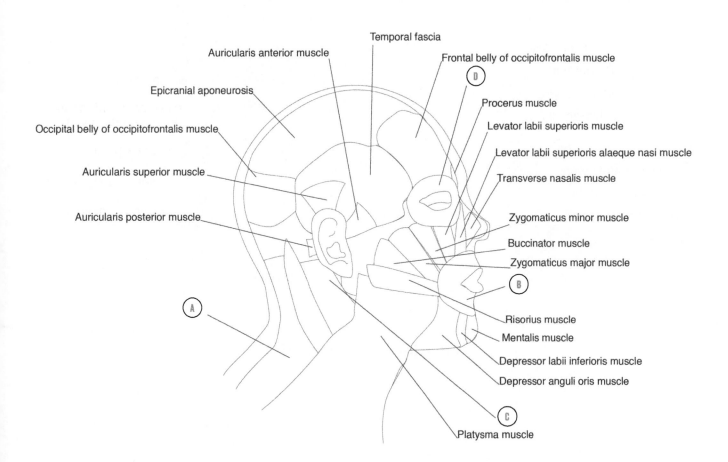

MUSCLES OF THE UPPER LIMBS

COLOURING NOTES 15.17

- ☐ Identify and label the biceps muscle. Colour it green.
- ☐ Identify and label the deltoid muscle. Colour it orange.
- ☐ Identify and label the flexor carpi radialis. Colour it brown.
- ☐ Identify and label the latissimus dorsi. Colour it pink.

- ☐ Identify and label the teres major muscle. Colour it purple.
- ☐ Identify and label the teres minor muscle. Colour it blue.
- ☐ Identify and label the trapezius muscle. Colour it yellow.
- ☐ Identify and label the triceps muscle. Colour it red.

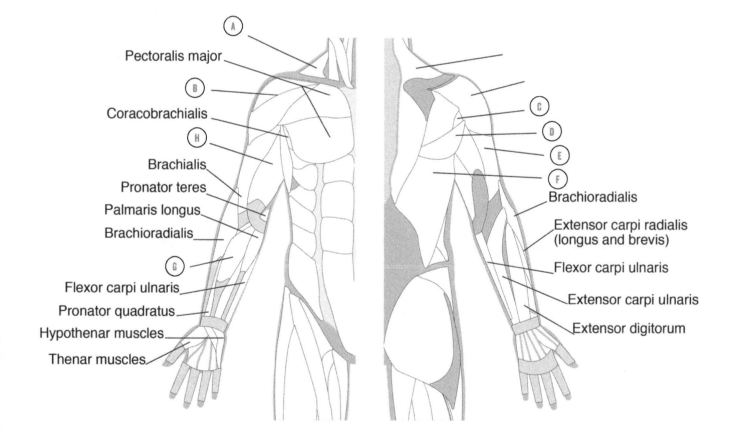

Pectoralis major

Coracobrachialis

Brachialis

Pronator teres

Palmaris longus

Brachioradialis

Flexor carpi ulnaris

Pronator quadratus

Hypothenar muscles

Thenar muscles

Brachioradialis

Extensor carpi radialis (longus and brevis)

Flexor carpi ulnaris

Extensor carpi ulnaris

Extensor digitorum

Anterior   **Posterior**

MUSCLES OF THE THORAX AND ABDOMEN (ANTERIOR VIEW)

COLOURING NOTES 15.18

- ☐ Identify and label the biceps brachii. Colour it yellow.
- ☐ Identify and label the deltoid muscle. Colour it orange.
- ☐ Identify and label the external abdominal oblique muscle. Colour it pink.
- ☐ Identify and label the internal abdominal oblique muscle. Colour it purple.
- ☐ Identify and label the pectoralis major muscle. Colour it brown.
- ☐ Identify and label the rectus abdominis. Colour it blue.
- ☐ Identify and label the trapezius muscle. Colour it green.

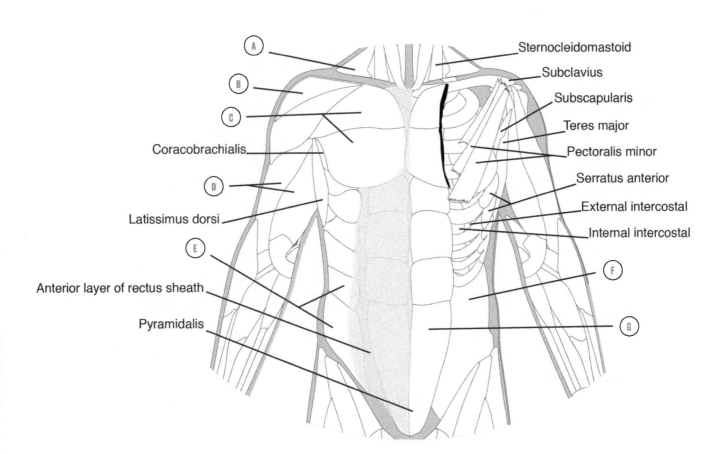

MUSCLES OF THE LEGS

COLOURING NOTES 15.19

- [ ] Identify and label both biceps femori muscle. Colour them purple.
- [ ] Identify and label the calcaneus (Achilles) tendon. Colour it brown.
- [ ] Identify and label the gastrocnemius muscle. Colour it pink.
- [ ] Identify and label the gluteus maximus muscle. Colour it red.

- [ ] Identify and label the rectus femoris muscle. Colour it orange.
- [ ] Identify and label the tibialis anterior muscle. Colour it green.
- [ ] Identify and label the vastus lateralis muscle. Colour it yellow.
- [ ] Identify and label the vastus medialis muscle. Colour it blue.

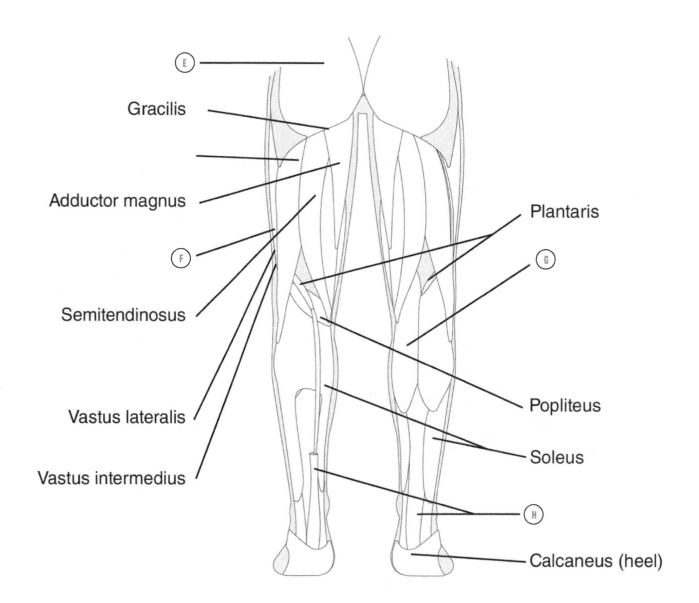

E

Gracilis

Adductor magnus

F

Semitendinosus

Vastus lateralis

Vastus intermedius

Plantaris

G

Popliteus

Soleus

H

Calcaneus (heel)

Posterior

MUSCLES OF THE LEGS (CONTINUED)

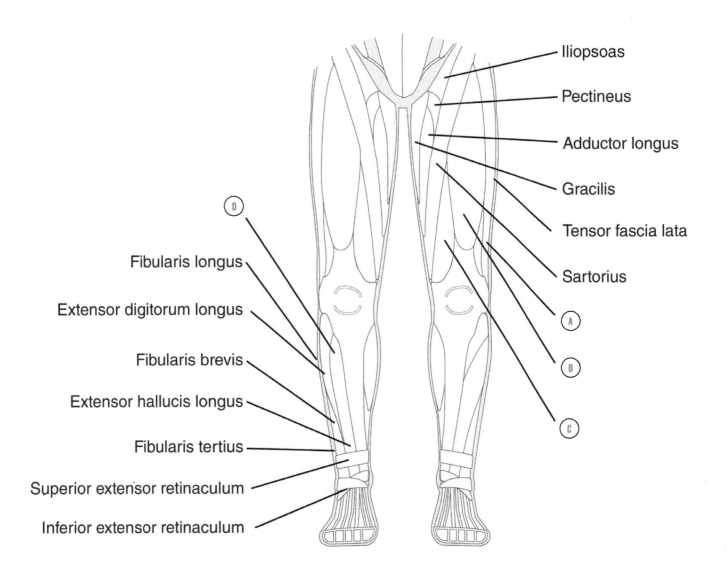

Iliopsoas

Pectineus

Adductor longus

Gracilis

Tensor fascia lata

Sartorius

Ⓐ

Ⓑ

Ⓒ

Ⓓ

Fibularis longus

Extensor digitorum longus

Fibularis brevis

Extensor hallucis longus

Fibularis tertius

Superior extensor retinaculum

Inferior extensor retinaculum

Anterior

CHAPTER 16

THE REPRODUCTIVE SYSTEMS

INTRODUCTION

Reproduction is fundamental to the biological need for sustaining life as well as the personal need to create and nurture. This chapter will help you to review the structure of the male and female reproductive systems with reference to their development through life, their function in conception, maternal changes during pregnancy and delivery, and nurturing of the infant after birth. Remember to revise Chapter 16 in *Essentials of Anatomy and Physiology for Nursing Practice*.

Answers to the labelling exercises can be found at the back of the book.

CROSS-SECTION OF THE SEMINIFEROUS TUBULE

INTRODUCTION

Male external genitalia develop during the third and fourth months of gestation and the foetus continues to grow, develop and differentiate. Testosterone produced from Leydig cells in the primitive testes furthers the formation of the male reproductive system through further differentiation of Wolffian ducts and common primordial genital tissue. Testosterone and Müllerian-Inhibiting Factor (MIF) secreted from immature Sertoli cells both inhibit differentiation of the Müllerian ducts into the female reproductive system.

COLOURING NOTES 16.1

- ☐ Identify and label the basement membrane.
- ☐ Identify and label the capillaries. Colour them red.
- ☐ Identify and label the developing sperm cells. Colour them pink.
- ☐ Identify and label the fibroblasts. Colour them grey.
- ☐ Identify and label the Leydig cells. Colour them green.
- ☐ Identify and label the lumen of the seminiferous tubule.

- ☐ Identify and label the Sertoli cells. Colour them purple.
- ☐ Identify and label the spermatids. Colour them yellow.
- ☐ Identify and label the spermatozoa. Colour them blue.
- ☐ Identify and label the tight junction between the Sertoli cells.

See p. 464 of *Essentials of Anatomy and Physiology for Nursing Practice* to check the answers.

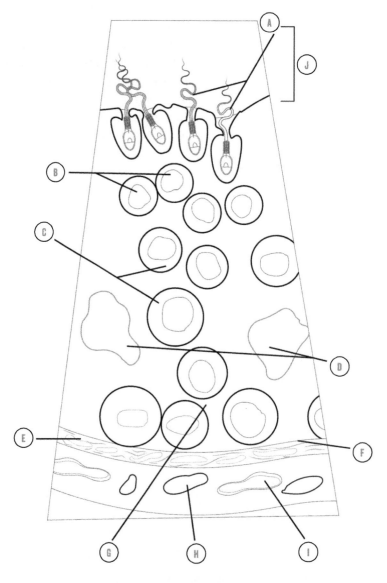

ANATOMY OF THE MALE REPRODUCTIVE SYSTEM

INTRODUCTION

The functions of the male reproductive system are:

- To form the male gametes (sperm) and male hormones (testosterone).
- To carry the sperm through the tubules for activation.
- To penetrate the female and deposit sperm within the female reproductive system.

COLOURING NOTES 16.2

- ☐ Identify and label the ampulla.
- ☐ Identify and label the bladder. Colour it yellow.
- ☐ Identify and label the bulbourethral gland. Colour it purple.
- ☐ Identify and label the ejaculatory duct and ductus deferens (vas deferens). Colour them blue.
- ☐ Identify and label the epididymis. Colour it orange.

- ☐ Identify and label the glans penis. Colour it pink.
- ☐ Identify and label the penis. Colour it grey.
- ☐ Identify and label the prostate gland. Colour it brown.
- ☐ Identify and label the scrotum.
- ☐ Identify and label the seminal vesicle. Colour it green.
- ☐ Identify and label the testis. Colour it red.
- ☐ Identify and label the urethra. Colour it yellow.

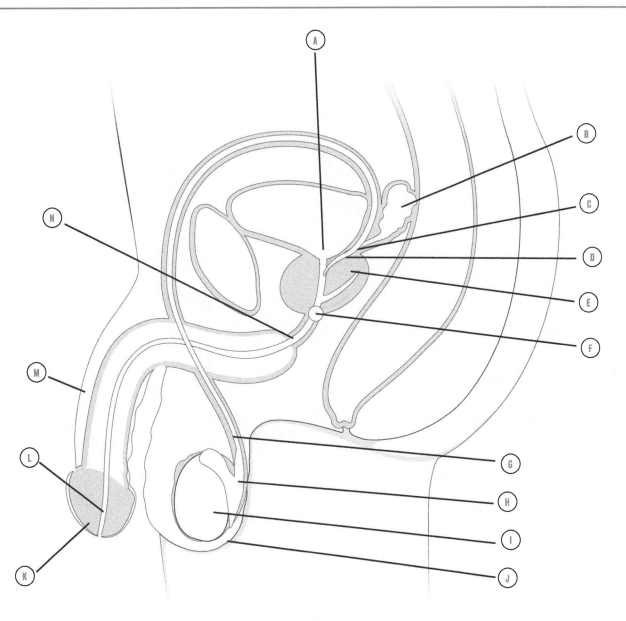

A TESTIS

INTRODUCTION

The testes are the reproductive glands which form the sperm and are oval in shape, 4–5 cm (2 inches) in length and 2.5 cm (1 inch) in diameter. The testes initially form within the abdomen but usually descend into the scrotum through the inguinal canal by the time of birth. They are suspended in the scrotum by the spermatic cord and the scrotum hangs outside the body, maintaining the testes at a temperature 1–2°C lower than core body temperature.

COLOURING NOTES 16.3

☐ Identify and label the:
- ○ Body of epididymis
- ○ Efferent ductule
- ○ Head of epididymis
- ○ Rete testis
- ○ Tail of epididymis.

☐ Colour the epididymis green.
☐ Identify and label the seminiferous tubule. Colour it yellow.
☐ Identify and label the tubulus rectus. Colour it yellow.

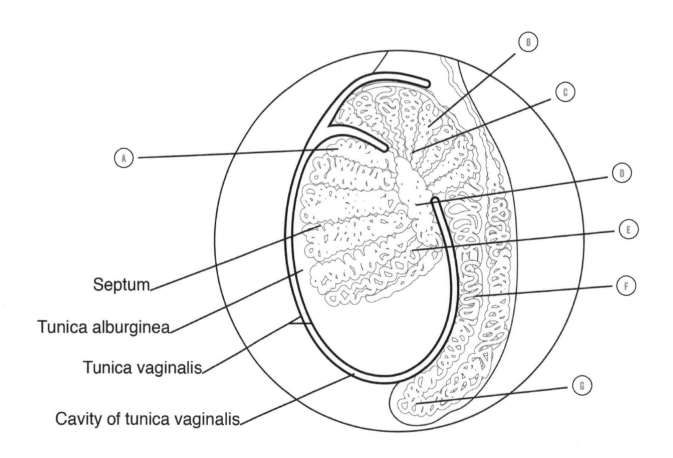

Septum

Tunica alburginea

Tunica vaginalis

Cavity of tunica vaginalis

A SPERM CELL

INTRODUCTION

Each testis contains about 200–300 lobules of which each contains 1–4 seminiferous tubules which produce sperm (spermatozoa) from germinal epithelial cells. Sperm are tiny cells that have three main sections:

1. The head.
2. The mid-piece.
3. The tail.

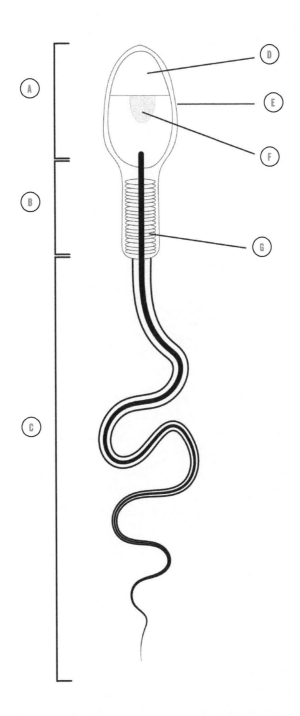

THE PENIS

INTRODUCTION

The penis is a tubular organ which anatomically consists of two halves: the root and the shaft and glans. The root is the internal attachment to the body wall and the shaft and glans make up the externally visible components of the penis. The urethra exits at the glans through the urethral meatus.

COLOURING NOTES 16.5

☐ Identify and label the bulb. Colour it light blue.
☐ Identify and label the corpus cavernosa. Colour it purple.
☐ Identify and label the corpus spongiosum. Colour it red.
☐ Identify and label the crura. Colour it dark blue.
☐ Identify and label the external urethral meatus.

☐ Identify and label the urethra. Colour it yellow.
☐ Identify and label the:

- Glans
- Neck
- Penile body (shaft)
- Prepuce
- Root.

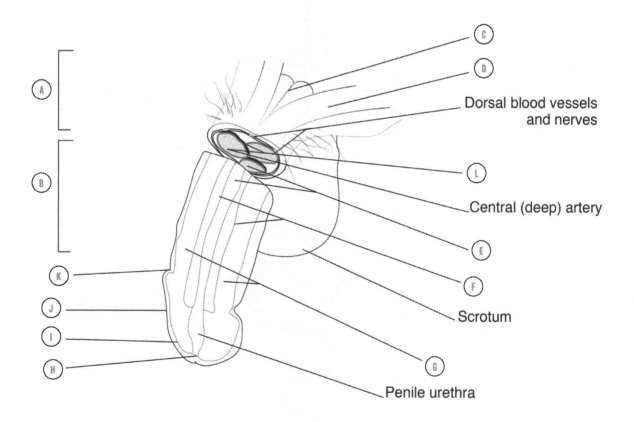

Dorsal blood vessels and nerves

Central (deep) artery

Scrotum

Penile urethra

ANATOMY OF THE FEMALE REPRODUCTIVE SYSTEM

INTRODUCTION

The female reproductive system develops from the Müllerian ducts. Parts of these fuse to form the uterus and vagina and the fused medial walls are resorbed from below upwards. The vagina develops from a rod of epithelial cells and the vagina forms as the centre of this rod breaks down. Development is complete by about the 20th week of gestation. The female reproductive organs are mainly internal.

The functions of the female reproductive system are to:

- Produce the female gametes, the ova.
- Transport the ovum along the Fallopian tube where it is fertilised.
- Protect and nurture the developing embryo and foetus until ready for birth.
- Deliver the baby safely.

ANATOMY OF THE FEMALE REPRODUCTIVE SYSTEM (ANTERIOR VIEW)

COLOURING NOTES 16.6

- ☐ Identify and label the cavity of the uterus. Colour it pink.
- ☐ Identify and label the cervix.
- ☐ Identify and label the fallopian tube. Colour it red.
- ☐ Identify and label the internal and external os.

- ☐ Identify and label the labium minus.
- ☐ Identify and label the muscle wall of the uterus. Colour it brown.
- ☐ Identify and label an ovary. Colour both orange.
- ☐ Identify and label the vagina. Colour it yellow.

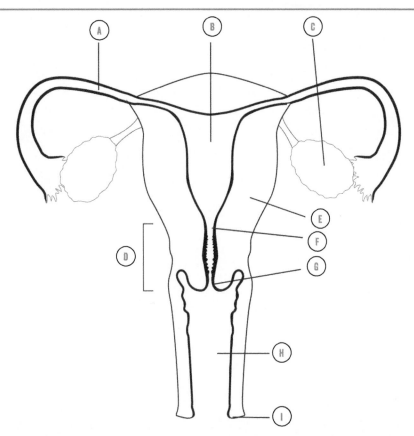

ANATOMY OF THE FEMALE REPRODUCTIVE SYSTEM (SAGITTAL SECTION)

COLOURING NOTES 16.7

☐ Identify and label the bladder. Colour it purple.
☐ Identify and label the cervical canal.
☐ Identify and label the clitoris.
☐ Identify and label the Fallopian tube. Colour it brown.
☐ Identify and label the labium minus and labium major.
☐ Identify and label the ovary. Colour it pink.

☐ Identify and label the rectum. Colour it green.
☐ Identify and label the symphysis pubis. Colour it light blue.
☐ Identify and label the urethra. Colour it orange.
☐ Identify and label the uterus. Colour it red.
☐ Identify and label the vagina. Colour it yellow.

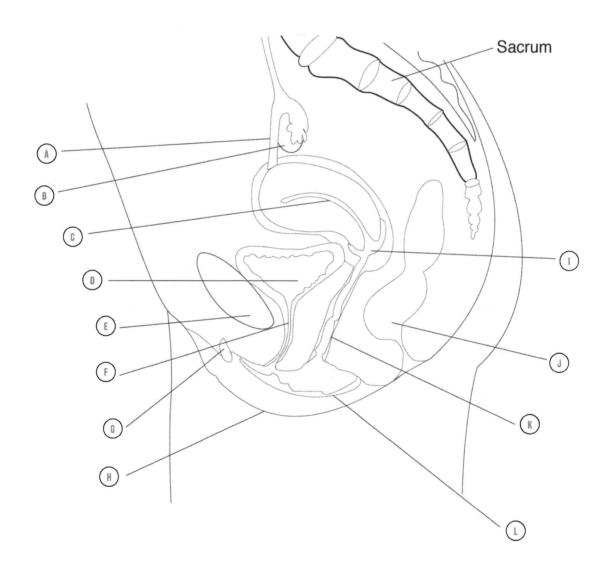

Sacrum

A
B
C
D
E
F
G
H
I
J
K
L

THE EXTERNAL FEMALE GENITALIA (VULVA)

COLOURING NOTES 16.8

☐ Identify and label the:

- Glans of clitoris
- Labia majora
- Labia minora
- Mons pubis
- Urethral opening.

☐ Identify and label the anus. Colour it grey.
☐ Identify and label the hymen. Colour it red.
☐ Identify and label the perineum. Colour it brown.
☐ Identify and label the prepuce of clitoris. Colour it orange.
☐ Identify and label the vestibule. Colour it yellow.

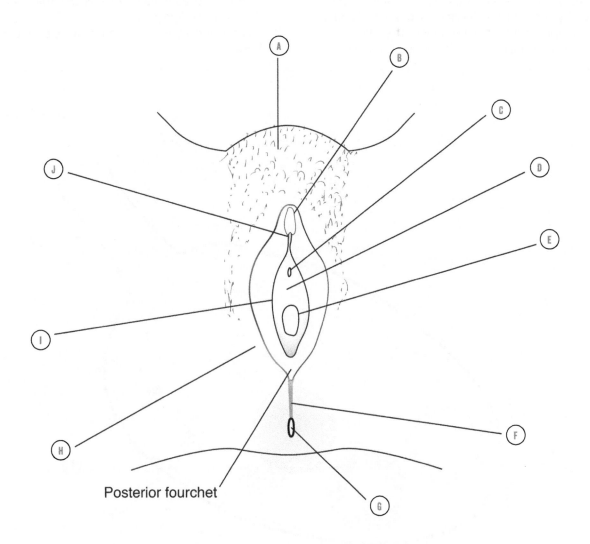

Posterior fourchet

OVARY ILLUSTRATING DEVELOPMENT OF OVUM AND CORPUS LUTEUM

INTRODUCTION

The ovaries in the female produce the female gametes and sex hormones. Primordial ova are present in the ovary at the birth of a baby girl, but development is halted until puberty when further development takes place to form the mature ovum. Maturation of the ovum takes place in the ovary, followed by ovulation and development of the corpus luteum. Ovarian follicles and corpora lutea (singular corpus luteum) both play an important role in the endocrine function of the ovaries.

COLOURING NOTES 16.9

- ☐ Identify and label the blood vessels. Colour them red.
- ☐ Identify and label the corona radiata. Shade it pink.
- ☐ Identify and label the developing, developed and degenerating corpora lutea. Colour them blue.
- ☐ Identify and label the oocyte. Colour it orange.

- ☐ Identify and label the ovulated ovum. Colour it purple.
- ☐ Identify and label the primordial and primary follicles. Colour them yellow.
- ☐ Identify and label the secondary follicle. Colour it brown.

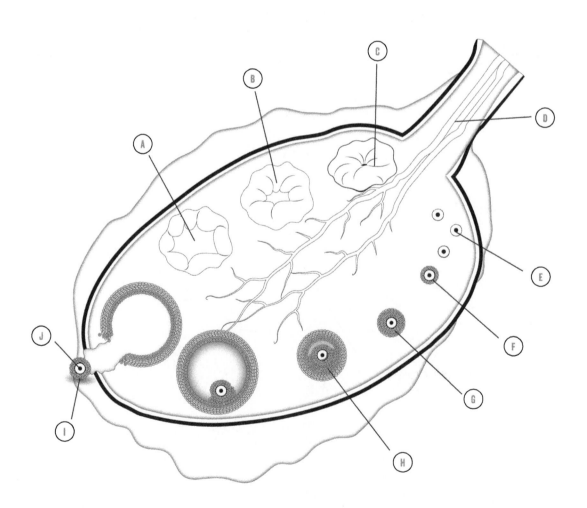

PREGNANCY AND GROWTH OF THE UTERUS

INTRODUCTION

Pregnancy usually lasts 38 weeks from the date of conception which, in someone with a regular four-weekly menstrual cycle, is 40 weeks after the first day of her last menstrual period. During that period the uterus grows to about 20 times its normal size. Normally it is about the fourth month before the mother can feel her baby moving. Towards the end of pregnancy, the baby normally takes up a head down position with the back towards the side and front of the woman's body and the head drops into the pelvis ready for a cephalic presentation birth – the most common position for delivery.

COLOURING NOTES 16.10

☐ Identify and label the bladder. Colour it yellow.
☐ Identify and label the rectum. Colour it blue.
☐ Identify and label the uterus. Colour it pink.
☐ Identify and label the vagina. Colour it green.

☐ Identify the vertebrae. Colour them orange.
☐ Identify where the uterus will have developed to at the third and seventh month of pregnancy.

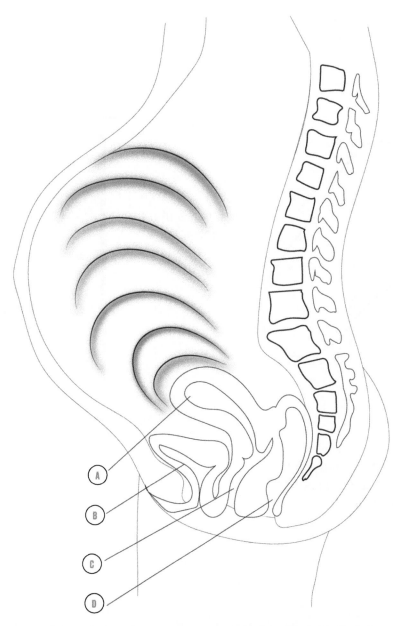

HORMONAL CONTROL OF LABOUR AND DELIVERY

INTRODUCTION

Towards the end of pregnancy the raised levels of oestrogen increase the numbers of oxytocin receptors in the uterus. Once labour starts, contractions cause cervical dilation which stimulates prostaglandin secretion and sends nerve impulses back to the brain. Positive feedback increases oxytocin, and causes yet more contractions. After delivery of the baby the presence of oxytocin stimulates uterine contractions and facilitates delivery of the placenta. It also promotes bonding by the mother with the baby.

COLOURING NOTES 16.11

- ☐ Fill in the three blanks with the correct hormones.
- ☐ Draw arrows to illustrate the positive feedback system and how the components interrelate.
- ☐ Colour the foetus pink.
- ☐ Colour the amniotic fluid yellow.
- ☐ Colour the uterine wall orange.

See p. 469 of *Essentials of Anatomy and Physiology for Nursing Practice* to check the answers.

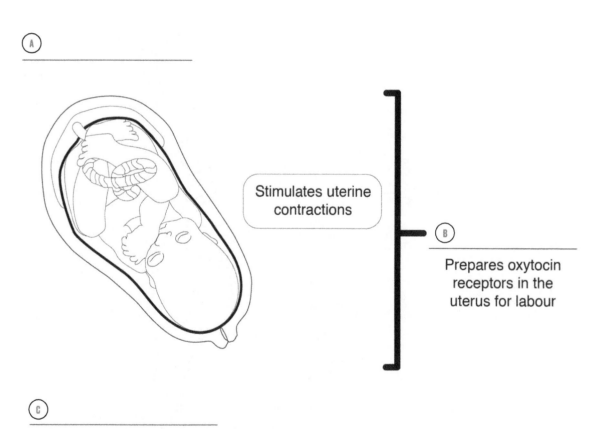

A _____

Stimulates uterine contractions

B _____
Prepares oxytocin receptors in the uterus for labour

C _____
From the foetus and maternal hypothalamus via the posterior pituitary gland

BREAST ANATOMY

INTRODUCTION

Under endocrine control during the second and third trimester of pregnancy, the breasts enlarge in preparation for breast-feeding the infant. Milk is stored in lactiferous sinuses prior to feeding.

COLOURING NOTES 16.12

- ☐ Identify and label the alveoli. Colour them grey.
- ☐ Identify and label the areola. Colour it brown.
- ☐ Identify and label the areolar glands.
- ☐ Identify and label the fat tissue. Colour it yellow.
- ☐ Identify and label the lactiferous ducts. Colour them green.
- ☐ Identify and label the lactiferous sinuses. Colour them blue.
- ☐ Identify and label the lobule. Colour them orange.
- ☐ Identify and label the nipple. Colour it pink.
- ☐ Identify and label the suspensory ligament.

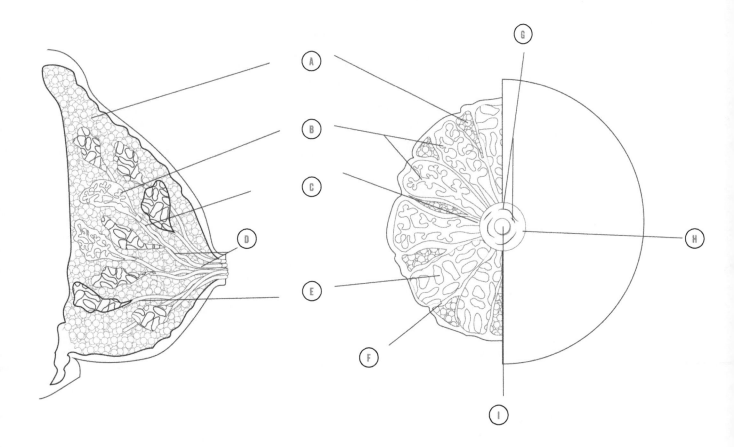

CHAPTER 17

DEVELOPMENT THROUGH THE LIFE SPAN

INTRODUCTION

Throughout life, from fertilisation of the egg to death, changes occur in the way in which the human body functions and thus in the requirements needed to maintain health. In order to meet the needs of individuals throughout their life span, you need to understand the stages in development including growth in size and increase in functional ability through childhood to adulthood, through activity in midlife, to diminution in height and reduced vitality in old age. This chapter will help you to review aspects of cell renewal and development. Remember to revise Chapter 17 in *Essentials of Anatomy and Physiology for Nursing Practice*.

Answers to the labelling exercises can be found at the back of the book.

APOPTOSIS

INTRODUCTION

Apoptosis is a major process in moving through the stages of development, removing cells and tissues no longer required and permitting remodelling. It can be genetically programmed or initiated by some external stresses such as hypoxia, nutrient deprivation, viral infection and/or damage to a cell membrane.

COLOURING NOTES 17.1

Please note the order of the stages of apoptosis have been jumbled up below.

☐ Identify and label the cells using the following headings:

- ○ Cell breaks apart
- ○ Cell damage or 'Death' signal
- ○ Cell shrinkage/blebbing
- ○ Macrophages remove parts

- ○ Normal cell
- ○ Nuclear collapse/signal macrophages.

☐ Colour the cytoplasm of the cells blue.
☐ Colour the nucleus of the normal cell green.
☐ Using arrows, indicate the order of the stages of cell apoptosis.

See p. 480 of *Essentials of Anatomy and Physiology for Nursing Practice* to check the answers.

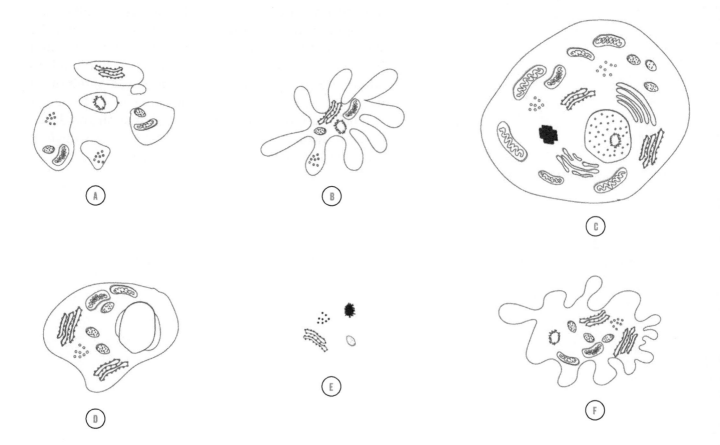

BLASTOCYST

INTRODUCTION

During the first eight weeks of development, growth is rapid and the basic structure of the human body is laid down. Fertilisation of the ovum by the sperm to form the zygote with a complete chromosome count of 46 takes place in the Fallopian tube and cell division begins. The small solid bunch of cells (morula) enters the uterus at about three days, develops a fluid-filled space, and is now referred to as a blastocyst. This embeds in the uterine wall at about seven days.

--- **COLOURING NOTES 17.2** ---

- ☐ Colour the cytoplasm of the cells blue and the nuclei green. Outline each cell in black.
- ☐ Colour the wall of the blastocyst purple.
- ☐ Identify and label the blastocyst cavity. Colour it yellow.
- ☐ Identify and label the inner cell mass.
- ☐ Identify and label the trophoblast.

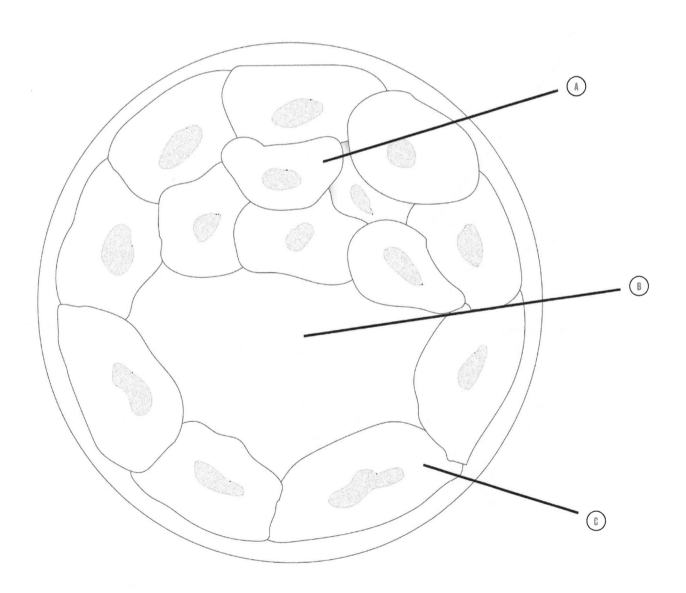

GASTRULATION STAGE: THREE GERM LAYERS

INTRODUCTION

Following implantation of the blastocyst in the uterine wall, gastrulation occurs when the three germ layers of the embryo form and the embryo develops a head-to-tail and front-to-back orientation.

COLOURING NOTES 17.3

☐ Identify and label the amniotic cavity. Colour it blue.
☐ Identify and label the chorion. Colour it grey.
☐ Identify and label the ectoderm layer. Colour it purple.
☐ Identify and label the endoderm layer. Colour it yellow.
☐ Identify and label the endometrium. Colour it pink.

☐ Identify and label the maternal blood pool. Colour it orange.
☐ Identify and label the mesoderm layer. Colour it orange.
☐ Identify and label the yolk sac. Colour it yellow.

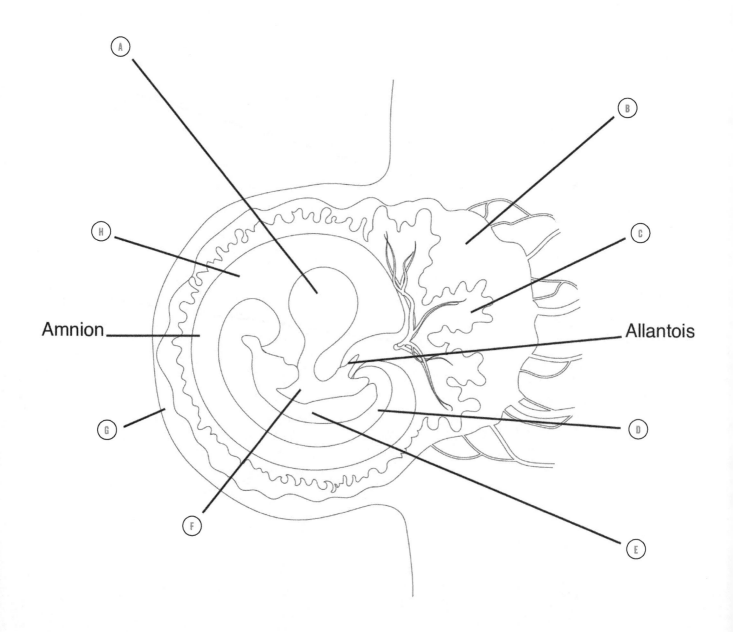

Amnion

Allantois

THE PLACENTA

INTRODUCTION

The placenta is also an endocrine organ, producing human chorionic gonadotrophin during early pregnancy. The placenta is mainly established by the fourth week of pregnancy, although it continues to develop through pregnancy. It is formed by both embryonic and maternal cells and the blood vessels of the two separate individuals are close but not linked to each other, permitting exchange of substances, but minimal cells, between the two circulations. During intrauterine life, the foetus obtains nutrients and oxygen from the mother and waste products are eliminated through the placenta into the maternal circulation from which they are excreted.

COLOURING NOTES 17.4

- ☐ Colour the umbilical vein red and the umbilical arteries blue.
- ☐ Identify and label the foetal capillaries.
- ☐ Identify and label the maternal arterioles. Colour them red.

- ☐ Identify and label the maternal venule. Colour it blue.
- ☐ Identify and label the placenta and uterine endometrium.
- ☐ Identify and label the umbilical cord.

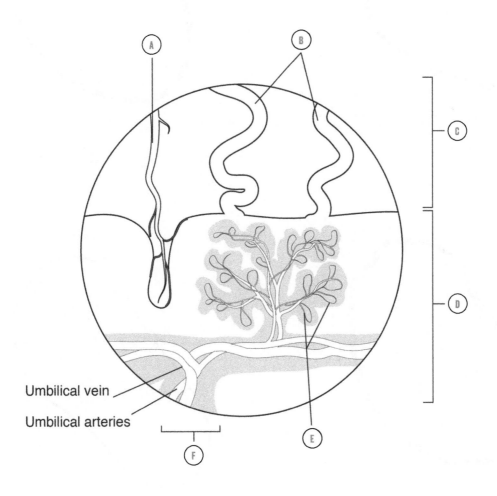

Umbilical vein
Umbilical arteries

THE DEVELOPING BABY THROUGH PREGNANCY

INTRODUCTION

During foetal development rapid growth and differentiation occur; the organs and systems develop in size and complexity to achieve readiness for beginning life after birth.

COLOURING NOTES 17.5

- ☐ Colour the amniotic fluid orange.
- ☐ Colour the foetus yellow.
- ☐ Colour the placenta pink.
- ☐ Colour the umbilical cord purple.

- ☐ Colour the uterus blue.
- ☐ Under each image, identify the stage of development in weeks and in months.

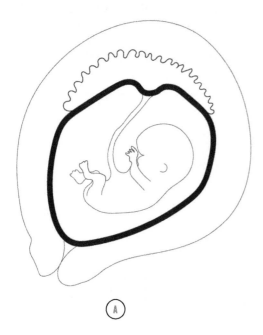

A

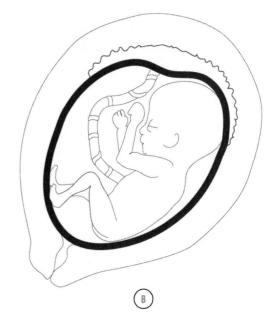

B

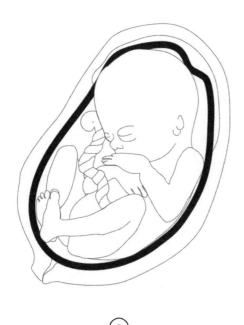

C

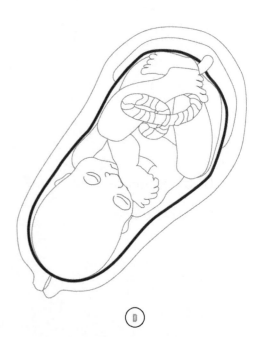

D

CARDIAC CHANGES FOLLOWING BIRTH

INTRODUCTION

In utero, the lungs are non-functional and the heart and circulation enable most of the blood to bypass the lungs. At birth, changes must occur immediately to enable the lungs to inspire air and provide oxygen to the body. As the baby takes its first breath the lungs expand and changes occur in the circulation to enable adequate blood flow to the lungs.

COLOURING NOTES 17.6

☐ Using arrows, indicate the direction of blood flow into the foetal heart.
☐ Label each of the four chambers of the heart.
☐ Identify and label the:

  ○ Foramen ovale
  ○ Inferior vena cava

  ○ Pulmonary vein(s)
  ○ Superior vena cava.

☐ Shade the walls of the heart orange.
☐ Colour the atria pink and ventricles red.

See p. 484 of *Essentials of Anatomy and Physiology for Nursing Practice* to check the answers.

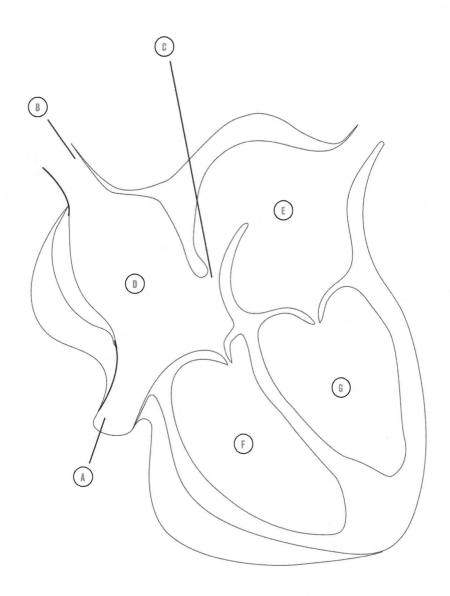

THE MATURE MALE AND FEMALE BODY

INTRODUCTION

Puberty usually starts earlier in girls than boys, with girls beginning puberty at 10–11 years old and completing it by 15–17, and boys beginning it at 11–12 and completing it by 16–17. Growth increases during the first half of puberty, with girls reaching their full height earlier than boys while skeletal changes result in the broad shoulders of young men, and the broad hips of women designed to facilitate childbirth. Growth of body hair and enlargement of the Adam's apple (angle of the thyroid cartilage in front of the larynx) in young men result in the characteristic male body and deeper voice.

COLOURING NOTES 17.7

☐ Choose a colour for the hair in each image and apply it. Shade the skin in both images in pink.
☐ Identify and label the following in the appropriate places:
  ○ Broad shoulders
  ○ Broader hips
  ○ Enlarged Adam's apple
  ○ Facial hair

○ Increased body hair
○ Increased musculature
○ Mature breasts
○ Mature genital organs
○ Pubic hair.

See p. 491 of *Essentials of Anatomy and Physiology for Nursing Practice* to check the answers.

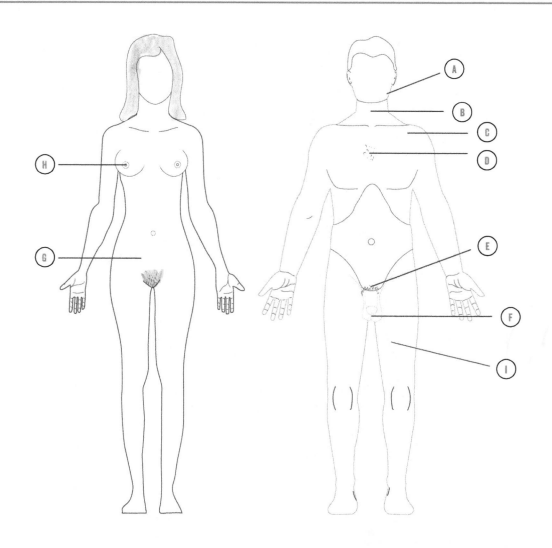

Female   **Male**

ANSWERS TO LABELLING EXERCISES

COLOURING NOTES 1.1

A. Chest
B. Cubital fossa
C. Umbilicus
D. Abdomen
E. Hip
F. Wrist
G. Palm
H. Knee
I. Heel
J. Foot
K. Left shoulder
L. Left arm
M. Left forearm
N. Left hand
O. Left thigh
P. Left lower leg

COLOURING NOTES 1.2

A. Left shoulder
B. Left elbow
C. Loin
D. Left buttock
E. Thigh
F. Left popliteal fossa
G. Left calf
H. Ankle
I. Heel

COLOURING NOTES 1.3

A. Superior
B. Proximal
C. Distal
D. Medial
E. Lateral
F. Inferior

COLOURING NOTES 1.5

A. Dorsal cavity
B. Spinal cavity
C. Cranial cavity

D. Thoracic cavity
E. Diaphragm
F. Abdominal cavity
G. Pelvic cavity
H. Abdominopelvic cavity
I. Ventral cavity

COLOURING NOTES 2.1

A. Macro context
B. Prerequisites
C. The care environment

COLOURING NOTES 2.2

A. Person-centred processes
B. Person-centred outcomes

COLOURING NOTES 2.3

A. Endocrine system
B. Gastrointestinal system
C. Respiratory system
D. Renal system
E. Cardiovascular system
F. Nervous system
G. Immune system
H. Integument
I. Musculoskeletal system
J. Skeletal system
K. Muscular system
L. Reproductive system

COLOURING NOTES 3.1

A. Secretory granules
B. Golgi apparatus
C. Rough endoplasmic reticulum
D. Nucleolus
E. Nuclear membrane
F. Nucleus
G. Smooth endoplasmic reticulum
H. Cell membrane
I. Centrioles
J. Centrosome

K. Mitochondrion
L. Ribosomes

COLOURING NOTES 3.3

A. Ribosome
B. Amino acids forming a protein chain
C. Nuclear membrane
D. Nuclear pore
E. Nucleus
F. DNA
G. mRNA

COLOURING NOTES 3.4

A. Intrinsic membrane proteins
B. Carbohydrate chain

COLOURING NOTES 3.5

A. Carrier protein
B. Amino acids, sugars, small proteins

COLOURING NOTES 3.7

A. Homologous chromosome
B. Sister chromatids
C. Homologues separate, sisters remain attached
D. Sisters separate
E. DNA Replication recombination
F. Chromosome segregation (meiosis I)
G. Chromosome segregation (meiosis II)
H. Gametes

COLOURING NOTES 3.8

A. Interphase
B. Prophase
C. Metaphase
D. Anaphase
E. Telophase
F. Homologous chromosome
G. Homologous chromosome
H. Chromatids separate

COLOURING NOTES 3.9

A. Chondrocytes
B. Collagen fibre
C. Elastic fibres
D. Chondrocytes
E. Chondrocytes

F. Cell nest
G. Solid matrix
H. Fibrocartilage
I. Elastic fibrocartilage
J. Hyaline

COLOURING NOTES 4.1

A. Flagellum
B. Cell wall
C. Pilus
D. DNA
E. Ribosomes
F. Cytoplasmic membrane
G. Cytoplasm

COLOURING NOTES 4.2

A. Single coccus
B. Staphylococci
C. Streptococci
D. Diplococci
E. Single bacillus
F. Coccobaclli
G. Vibrios
H. Spirochaetes

COLOURING NOTES 4.3

A. Diplococci
B. Flagellated bacteria
C. Bacillus with spores
D. Spores incorporated into chains
E. Fimbriated bacterium
F. Bacterium (bacillus)
G. Spores

COLOURING NOTES 4.4

A. Chromosome
B. Mother cell
C. Cell lengthens and duplicates its DNA
D. DNA molecules separate
E. Cross wall formation
F. Daughter cells

COLOURING NOTES 4.5

A. Protein coat
B. Nucleic acid
C. DNA
D. Tail (sheath)
E. Fibres

COLOURING NOTES 4.6

A. Protein coat
B. RNA
C. Membrane envelope

COLOURING NOTES 4.7

A. Virus capsule
B. Cell membrane
C. Cytoplasm
D. Cell nucleus containing DNA

COLOURING NOTES 4.8

A. Hyphae
B. Nucleus
C. Nucleus
D. Tough wall
E. Spore

COLOURING NOTES 4.9

A. Cilia
B. Pseudopod
C. Flagellum
D. Paramecium
E. Amoeba
F. Euglena

COLOURING NOTES 4.10

A. Mouth
B. Testis
C. Intestine
D. Ovary
E. Anus

COLOURING NOTES 4.11

A. Hooks
B. Sucker
C. Head
D. Neck
E. Tapes

COLOURING NOTES 4.12

A. *Gut-brain* autism, mood depression, anxiety
B. *Hypertension,* ischaemic heart disease
C. *Asthma/allergy*
D. *Altered drug metabolism*
E. *Obesity/metabolic syndrome,* altered energy/ lipid metabolism, diabetes

F. *Gall-bladder* bile circulation
G. *Colon cancer,* diet high in red mead and animal fat, low SCFA/butyrate, low vitamin absorption, low in sulphur metabolising bacteria. *Inflammatory bowel disease,* hygiene hypothesis, altered immune response, less microbial diversity

COLOURING NOTES 4.13

A. Epidermis
B. Dermis

COLOURING NOTES 5.1

A. Neurofibrils
B. Axon
C. Node of Ranvier
D. Dendrites
E. Nucleus
F. Axon terminal

COLOURING NOTES 5.2

A. Presynaptic neuron
B. Postsynaptic neuron
C. Presynaptic membrane
D. Gap junction
E. Postsynaptic membrane

COLOURING NOTES 5.3

A. Axon
B. Synaptic vesicle
C. Dendrite
D. Synaptic cleft
E. Neurotransmitter
F. Receptor site
G. Mitochondrion

COLOURING NOTES 5.4

A. Thalamus
B. Hypothalamus
C. Cerebellum
D. Pons
E. Medulla oblongata
F. Pituitary gland

COLOURING NOTES 5.5

A. Frontal lobe
B. Parietal lobe

C. Occipital lobe
D. Temporal lobe

COLOURING 5.6

A. Grey matter
B. White matter
C. Interneuron

COLOURING 5.7

A. Third-order neuron
B. Second-order neuron
C. First-order neuron (afferent neuron)

COLOURING NOTES 5.8

A. Sensory neuron
B. Motor neuron
C. Interneuron

COLOURING NOTES 5.9

A. Cervical
B. Thoracic
C. Lumbar
D. Sacral
E. Coccygeal

COLOURING NOTES 5.10

A. Middle cerebral artery
B. Anterior communicating artery
C. Internal carotid arteries
D. Circle of Willis
E. Basilar artery
F. Vertebral artery

COLOURING NOTES 5.11

A. Fourth ventricle
B. Lateral ventricle
C. Third ventricle
D. Subarachnoid space
E. Cerebellum

COLOURING NOTES 5.12

A. Skull
B. Dura matter
C. Arachnoid mater
D. Pia mater

COLOURING NOTES 6.1

A. Posterior cavity
B. Sclera
C. Retina
D. Choroid
E. Optic disc
F. Ciliary body
G. Anterior cavity
H. Iris
I. Cornea
J. Pupil
K. Lens
L. Optic nerve

COLOURING NOTES 6.3

A. Circumvallate papillae
B. Filiform papillae
C. Foliate papillae
D. Fungiform papillae
E. Sweet
F. Salty
G. Sour
H. Bitter

COLOURING NOTES 6.4

A. Taste pore
B. Gustatory hair
C. Gustatory receptor cell
D. Basal cell
E. Sensory neurons
F. Connective tissue
G. Supporting cell

COLOURING NOTES 6.5

A. Olfactory bulb
B. Cribriform formina
C. Axon
D. Basal cell
E. Supporting cell
F. Olfactory neuron
G. Dendrite
H. Cilia
I. Olfactory vesicle

COLOURING NOTES 6.6

A. Auricle
B. Temporal bone
C. Tympanic membrane
D. Semi-circular canals
E. Oval window

F. Cochlea
G. Auditory tube
H. Stapes
I. Incus
J. Malleus
K. Earlobe
L. Auditory canal

COLOURING NOTES 6.7

A. Semi-circular canals
B. Utricle
C. Saccule
D. Auditory nerve
E. Cochlea
F. Oval window
G. Ampulla

COLOURING NOTES 6.8

A. Tactile corpuscles
B. Free nerve endings
C. Merkel cells
D. Tactile discs
E. Root hair plexus
F. Ruffini corpuscles
G. Lamellated corpuscles

COLOURING NOTES 7.1

A. Classical endocrine
B. Paracrine
C. Autocrine
D. Intracine
E. Juxtacrine

COLOURING NOTES 7.2

A. Hypothalamus
B. Pineal
C. Pituitary
D. Thyroid
E. Parathyroid
F. Thymus
G. Pancreas
H. Adrenal glands
I. Ovaries
J. Testes

COLOURING NOTES 7.3

A. Thalamus
B. Pineal gland
C. Pituitary gland
D. Hypothalamus

COLOURING NOTES 7.4

A. Thyroid gland
B. Parathyroid glands

COLOURING NOTES 7.5

A. Zona glomerulosa
B. Zona fasciculata
C. Zona recticularis
D. Medulla

COLOURING NOTES 7.6

A. Beta (β) cell
B. Alpha (α) cell
C. Gamma (γ) cell
D. Blood capillaries

COLOURING NOTES 7.7

A. Afferent arteriole
B. Glomerular capsule
C. Efferent arteriole
D. Macula densa cells
E. Granular cells
F. Afferent arteriole
G. Red blood cells
H. Proximal tubule cells

COLOURING NOTES 8.1

A. Mouth
B. Oesophagus
C. Stomach
D. Pancreas
E. Large intestine
F. Small intestine
G. Rectum
H. Anus
I. End of small intestine
J. Beginning of large intestine
K. Duodenum
L. Gall bladder
M. Liver

COLOURING NOTES 8.2

A. Epithelium
B. Lamina propria
C. Muscularis mucosa
D. Submucosa
E. Circular layer
F. Outer longitudinal layer
G. Serosa
H. Mesentery

I. Lymph vessel
J. Vein
K. Artery
L. Villi

COLOURING NOTES 8.4

A. Enamel
B. Dentine
C. Pulp
D. Cementum
E. Nerves and blood vessels
F. Root end opening
G. Bone
H. Gums
I. Crown

COLOURING NOTES 8.5

A. Canine
B. Molars
C. Premolars
D. Incisors

COLOURING NOTES 8.6

A. Parotid glands
B. Parotid ducts
C. Sublingual duct
D. Sublingual glands
E. Submandibular duct
F. Submandibular glands

COLOURING NOTES 8.7

A. Oesophagus
B. Cardiac sphincter
C. Fundus
D. Body
E. Longitudinal muscle
F. Circular muscle
G. Oblique muscle
H. Rugae
I. Pyloric antrum
J. Duodenum
K. Pyloric sphincter

COLOURING NOTES 8.8

A. Villi
B. Intestinal glands
C. Lacteal (lymph vessel)

COLOURING NOTES 8.9

A. Transverse colon
B. Descending colon
C. Sigmoid colon
D. Rectum
E. Anus
F. Vermiform appendix
G. Caecum
H. Ascending colon

COLOURING NOTES 9.1

A. Falciform ligament
B. Right lobe
C. Left lobe
D. Gall bladder
E. Caudate lobe
F. Left lobe
G. Right lobe
H. Quadrate lobe
I. Gall bladder

COLOURING NOTES 9.2

A. Interlobular vein
B. Hepatic sinusoid
C. Hepatocyte
D. Central vein

COLOURING NOTES 9.3

A. Inferior vena cava
B. Hepatic vein
C. Right lobe
D. Left lobe
E. Hepatic artery
F. Portal vein
G. Aorta

COLOURING NOTES 10.1

A. Nasal cavities
B. Larynx
C. Trachea
D. Pulmonary vessels
E. Bronchi
F. Heart
G. Pleural membrane
H. Diaphragm
I. Pharynx
J. Epiglottis
K. Oesophagus

L. Intercostal muscles
M. Bronchioles
N. Alveoli

COLOURING NOTES 10.2

A. Frontal sinus
B. Nostril
C. Hard palate
D. Uvula
E. Tongue
F. Epiglottis
G. Trachea
H. Sphenoidal sinus
I. Nasopharynx
J. Palatine tonsil
K. Oropharynx
L. Lingual tonsil
M. Laryngopharynx
N. Oesophagus

COLOURING NOTES 10.3

A. Epiglottis
B. Cuneiform cartilage
C. Thyroid cartilage
D. Corniculate cartilage
E. Arytenoid cartilage
F. Cricoid cartilage
G. Cricothyroid ligament
H. Trachea

COLOURING NOTES 10.4

A. Trachea
B. Primary bronchus
C. Secondary bronchus
D. Tertiary bronchi
E. Bronchioles

COLOURING NOTES 10.5

A. Respiratory bronchiole
B. Deoxygenated blood from
   pulmonary artery
C. Oxygenated blood to pulmonary vein
D. Alveolus
E. Capillaries

COLOURING NOTES 10.6

A. Sternomastoid muscles
B. Scalene muscles
C. Inspiratory intercostal muscles

D. Expiratory intercostal muscles
E. Diaphragm
F. Pectoralis minor
G. Expiratory intercostal muscles
H. External oblique muscles
I. Expiratory abdominal muscles

COLOURING NOTES 10.7

A. Red blood cell
B. Tissue cells

COLOURING NOTES 11.4

A. Afferent arteriole
B. Glomerular capillary
C. Efferent arteriole
D. Bowman's capsule
E. Tubule

COLOURING NOTES 11.5

A. Adrenal glands
B. Kidneys
C. Ureters
D. Bladder
E. Urethra

COLOURING NOTES 11.6

A. Renal sinus
B. Adipose tissue
C. Renal pelvis
D. Renal papilla
E. Ureter
F. Cortex
G. Medulla
H. Renal pyramid
I. Minor calyx
J. Major calyx
K. Renal lobe
L. Renal columns
M. Renal capsule

COLOURING NOTES 11.7

A. Afferent arteriole
B. Efferent arteriole
C. Bownman's capsule
D. Glomerulus (capillaries)
E. Proximal convoluted tubule
F. Descending limb
G. Loop of Henle

H. Ascending limb
I. Distal convoluted tubule
J. Collecting duct

COLOURING NOTES 11.8

A. Ureters
B. Dome of fundus
C. Rugae
D. Ureteral orifice
E. Wall of bladder
F. Bladder neck
G. Urethra

COLOURING NOTES 12.1

A. Trachea
B. Oesophagus
C. Pulmonary artery
D. Pulmonary veins
E. Left lung
F. Heart
G. Diaphragm
H. Aorta
I. Inferior vena cava
J. Superior vena cava
K. Aorta
L. Clavicle

COLOURING NOTES 12.2

A. Pericardium
B. Fibrous layer
C. Parietal pericardium
D. Visceral pericardium
E. Myocardium
F. Endocardium

COLOURING NOTES 12.3

A. Aorta
B. Pulmonary artery
C. Left pulmonary vein
D. Left atrium
E. Mitral valve
F. Aortic valve
G. Pulmonary valve
H. Inferior vena cava
I. Tricuspid valve
J. Right atrium
K. Right pulmonary vein
L. Superior vena cava
M. Right ventricle
N. Left ventricle

COLOURING NOTES 12.4

A. Circumflex artery
B. Great cardiac vein
C. Anterior interventricular artery
D. Marginal artery
E. Anterior cardiac veins
F. Right coronary artery

COLOURING NOTES 12.5

A. External carotid
B. Left common carotid
C. Aorta
D. Ulnar
E. Radial
F. Dorsal pedis
G. Posterial tibial
H. Anterior tibial
I. Popliteal
J. Femoral
K. Abdominal aorta
L. Brachial
M. Axilliary
N. Right common carotid
O. Internal carotid

COLOURING NOTES 12.6

A. External jugular
B. Internal jugular
C. Axilliary
D. Cephalic
E. Brachial
F. Subclavian
G. Great saphenous
H. Small saphenous

COLOURING NOTES 12.7

A. Lumen
B. Tunica intima
C. Tunica media
D. Tunica externa
D. Artery
F. Vein

COLOURING NOTES 12.8

A. Valve closed
B. Valve cusp
C. Valve opened

COLOURING NOTES 12.9

A. Capillary wall
B. Cells
C. Venule
D. Vein
E. Artery
F. Arteriole

COLOURING NOTES 12.10

A. Left lymphatic duct
B. Thoracic duct
C. Lumbar lymph nodes
D. Popliteal lymph nodes
E. Inguinal lymph nodes
F. Axilliary lymph nodes
G. Thoracic lymph nodes
H. Right lymphatic duct
I. Cervical lymph nodes

COLOURING NOTES 12.13

A. Left atrium
B. Left ventricle
C. Bundle branches
D. Purkinje fibres
E. Right ventricle
F. Atrioventricular bundle
G. Atrioventricular node
H. Right atrium
I. Sinoatrial node

COLOURING NOTES 13.1

A. *Nasal cavity*: Particles filtered from air by cilia and trapped in mucus
B. *Bronchi*: Further filtering of particles from the air by cilia and trapped in mucus for removal
C. *Stomach*: Acidic hydrochloric acid kills pathogens
D. *GIT*: Intestinal microbiota stimulate lymphoid tissue within the gut mucosa to produce antibodies to pathogens
E. *Small intestine*: Lymphoid tissue (Peyer's patches) in lower part contributes to keeping microbes under control
F. *Vagina*: Acidic end products of commensals prevent colonisation by pathogens
G. *Skin*: Keratinised cells provide a physical barrier to pathogens, Commensals, end products of metabolism and antimicrobial lysozyme prevent pathogens colonising

H. *Pharynx:* Cilia move particles up the respiratory tract, mucus traps them and phagocytes destroys them
I. *Eyes*: Antimicrobial lysozymes in tears prevents pathogen colonisation

COLOURING NOTES 13.2

A. Thymus
B. Spleen
C. Bone marrow

COLOURING NOTES 14.1

A. Sweat pore
B. Hair shaft
C. Tactile corpuscle
D. Hair follicle
E. Sebaceous gland
F. Nerve fibre
G. Lamellated corpuscle
H. Arrector pilli muscle
I. Sweat gland
J. Hypodermis
K. Dermis
L. Epidermis
M. Papillary layer
N. Reticular layer

COLOURING NOTES 14.2

A. Fibroblast
B. Neutrophil
C. Platelet
D. Capillary
E. Epithelial cells
F. Eschar
G. New blood vessels
H. Granulation tissue
I. Neutrophils
J. Fibroblast

COLOURING NOTES 15.1

A. Clavical
B. Scapula
C. Sternum
D. Rib
E. Humerus
F. Vertebrae
G. Radius
H. ulna
I. Carpals

J. Metacarpals
K. Phalanges
L. Pelvis
M. Femur
N. Patella
O. Tibia
P. Fibula
Q. Tarsals
R. Metatarsals
S. Phalanges

COLOURING NOTES 15.2

A. Epiphysis
B. Diaphysis
C. Epiphysis
D. Articular cartilage
E. Epiphyseal line
F. Spongy bone
G. Medullary cavity
H. Nutrient foramen
I. Endosteum
J. Periosteum
K. Articular cartilage

COLOURING NOTES 15.3

A. Osteon
B. Circumferential lamellae
C. Blood vessels within central canal
D. Osteocytes in lacunae
E. Blood vessels within perforating canal
F. Periosteum
G. Interstitial lamellae
H. Concentric lamellae

COLOURING NOTES 15.4

A. Trabeculae
B. Spaces containing bone marrow and blood vessels

COLOURING NOTES 15.5

A. Sutural bone
B. Flat bone
C. Long bone
D. Short bones
E. Irregular bone
F. Sesamoid bone

COLOURING NOTES 15.6

A. Frontal bone
B. Parietal bone

C. Occipital bone
D. Temporal bone
E. Ethmoid bone
F. Sphenoid bone

COLOURING NOTES 15.7

A. Frontal bone
B. Nasal bone (2)
C. Perpendicular plate of ethmoid (1)
D. Vomer (1)
E. Mandible (1)
F. Inferior nasal concha (2)
G. Maxilla (2)
H. Zygomatic bone (2)
I. Lacrimal bone (2)
J. Palatine bone (2)

COLOURING NOTES 15.8

A. Spinous process
B. Transverse processes
C. Pedicles
D. Space for spinal cord
E. Vertebral body

COLOURING NOTES 15.9

A. Cervical vertebrae
B. Thoracic vertebrae
C. Lumbar vertebrae
D. Sacral vertebrae
E. Coccygeal vertebrae

COLOURING NOTES 15.10

A. True ribs (1-7)
B. False ribs (8-10)
C. Floating ribs (11-12)
D. Clavicular notch
E. Manubrium
F. Sternal angle
G. Body
H. Xiphoid process
I. Costal cartilage
J. Sternum

COLOURING NOTES 15.11

A. Pectoral girdle
B. Clavicle
C. Scapula
D. Humerus
E. Radius

F. Ulna
G. Carpals
H. Metacarpals
I. Phalanges

COLOURING NOTES 15.12

A. Sacrum
B. Ilium
C. Iliac crest
D. Coccyx
E. Acetabulum, *where femur articulates with pelvis*
F. Pubic crest
G. Pubic Symphysis
H. Pubic arch
I. Ischium
J. Pubic bone

COLOURING NOTES 15.13

A. Femur
B. Patella
C. Tibia
D. Fibula
E. Tarsals
F. Metatarsals
G. Phalanges

COLOURING NOTES 15.14

A. Bone
B. Synovial membrane
C. Articular cartilage
D. Joint cavity containing synovial fluid
E. Articular capsule

COLOURING NOTES 15.15

A. Actin myofilament
B. Myosin myofilament
C. Striations
D. Sarcomere
E. Myofibrils
F. Sarcolemma (cell membrane)
G. Nucleus
H. Capillary
I. Endomysium (between muscle fibres)
J. Fasciculi
K. Fascicle
L. Endomysium
M. Blood vessel
N. Epimysum

COLOURING NOTES 15.16

A. Trapezius muscle
B. Orbicularis oris
C. Sternocleidomastoid
D. Obicularis oculi

COLOURING 15.17

A. Trapezius
B. Deltoid
C. Teres minor
D. Teres major
E. Triceps
F. Latissimus dorsi
G. Flexor carpi radialis
H. Bicep

COLOURING NOTES 15.18

A. Trapezius
B. Deltoid
C. Pectoralis major
D. Biceps brachii
E. External abdominal oblique
F. Internal abdominal oblique
G. Rectus abdominis

COLOURING NOTES 15.19

A. Vastus lateralis
B. Rectus femoris
C. Vastus medialis
D. Tibalis anterior
E. Gluteus maximus
F. Biceps femoris
G. Gastrocnemius
H. Calcaneus (Achilles) tendon

COLOURING NOTES 16.1

A. Spermatozoa (mature sperm cells)
B. Spermatids
C. Developing sperms cells
D. Sertoli cells
E. Fibroblast
F. Basement membrane
G. Tight junction between sertoli cells
H. Leydig cells
I. Capillary
J. Lumen of the seminiferous tubule

COLOURING NOTES 16.2

A. Urinary bladder opening
B. Seminal vesicles

C. Ampulla
D. Ejaculatory duct
E. Prostate gland
F. Bulbourethral gland
G. Ductus deferens
H. Epididymis
I. Testis
J. Scrotum
K. Glans penis
L. Urethra
M. Penis
N. Membranous urethra

COLOURING NOTES 16.3

A. Seminiferous tubule
B. Head of epididymis
C. Efferent ductile
D. Rete testis
E. Tubulus rectus
F. Body of epididymis
G. Tail of epididymis

COLOURING NOTES 16.4

A. Head
B. Midipiece
C. Tail (flagellum)
D. Acrosome
E. Cell membrane
F. Nucleus
G. Mitochondria

COLOURING NOTES 16.5

A. Root
B. Body (shaft)
C. Bulb of penis
D. Crura of penis
E. Uretha
F. Corpus spongiosum
G. Corpus cavermosa
H. External urethral meatus
I. Glans
J. Prepuce (foreskin)
K. Neck
L. Corpus cavernosa

COLOURING NOTES 16.6

A. Fallopian tube
B. Cavity of uterus
C. Ovary
D. Cervix
E. Muscle wall of uterus

F. Internal OS
G. External OS
H. Vagina
I. Labium minus

COLOURING NOTES 16.7

A. Fallopian tube
B. Ovary
C. Uterus
D. Bladder
E. Symphysis pubis
F. Urethra
G. Clitoris
H. Labium major
I. Cervical canal
J. Rectum
K. Vagina
L. Labium minus

COLOURING NOTES 16.8

A. Mons pubis
B. Prepuce of clitoris
C. Urethral opening
D. Vestibule
E. Hymen
F. Perineum
G. Anus
H. Labia majora
I. Labia minora
J. Glans of clitoris

COLOURING NOTES 16.9

A. Developing corpus luteum
B. Corpus luteum
C. Degenerating corpus luteum
D. Ovarian blood vessels passing through the ovarian ligament
E. Primordial follicles
F. Primary follicles
G. Oocyte
H. Secondary follicle
I. Corona radiate
J. Ovulated ovum

COLOURING 16.10

A. Uterus
B. Bladder
C. Vagina
D. Rectum

COLOURING NOTES 16.11

A. Prostaglandins
B. Oestrogen
C. Oxytocin

COLOURING NOTES 16.12

A. Fat tissue
B. Alveoli
C. Lactiferous duct
D. Lactiferous sinuses
E. Lobule
F. Suspensory ligament
G. Areolar glands
H. Areola
I. Nipple

COLOURING NOTES 17.1

A. Cell breaks apart
B. Nuclear collapse/signal macrophages
C. Normal cell
D. Cell damage
E. Macrophages remove parts
F. Cell shrinkage/blebbing

COLOURING NOTES 17.2

A. Inner cell mass
B. Blastocyst cavity
C. Trophoblast

COLOURING NOTES 17.3

A. Yolk sac
B. Maternal blood pool
C. Chorion
D. Ectoderm layer
E. Mesoderm layer
F. Endoderm layer

G. Endometrium
H. Amniotic cavity

COLOURING NOTES 17.4

A. Maternal venule
B. Maternal arterioles
C. Uterine endometrium
D. Placenta
E. Foetal capillaries bathed in maternal blood
F. Umbilical cord

COLOURING NOTES 17.5

A. Month 3 (9-12 weeks)
B. Month 5 (17-20 weeks)
C. Month 7 (25-28 weeks)
D. Month 9 (33-36 weeks)

COLOURING NOTES 17.6

A. Inferior vena cava
B. Superior vena cava
C. Foramen ovale (closes after birth)
D. Right atrium
E. Left atrium
F. Right ventricle
G. Left ventricle

COLOURING NOTES 17.7

A. Facial hair
B. Enlarged Adam's apple
C. Broad shoulders
D. Increased body hair
E. Pubic hair
F. Mature genital organs
G. Broader hips
H. Mature breasts
I. Increased musculature

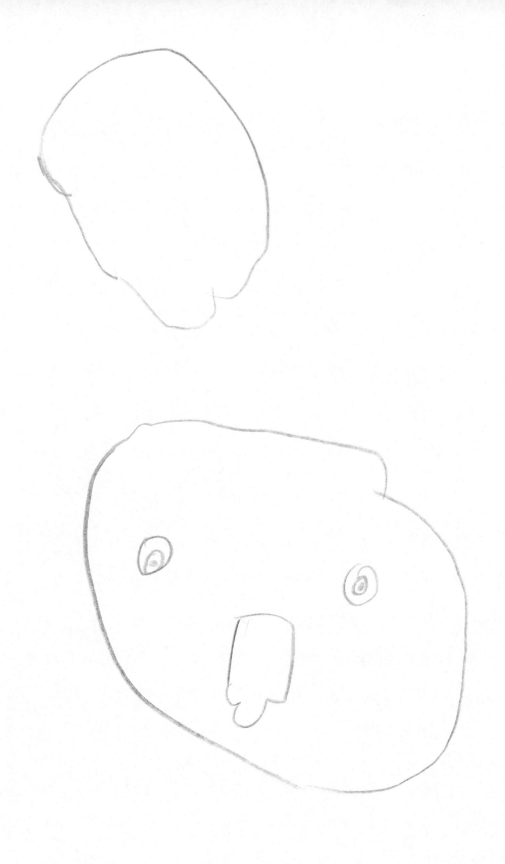

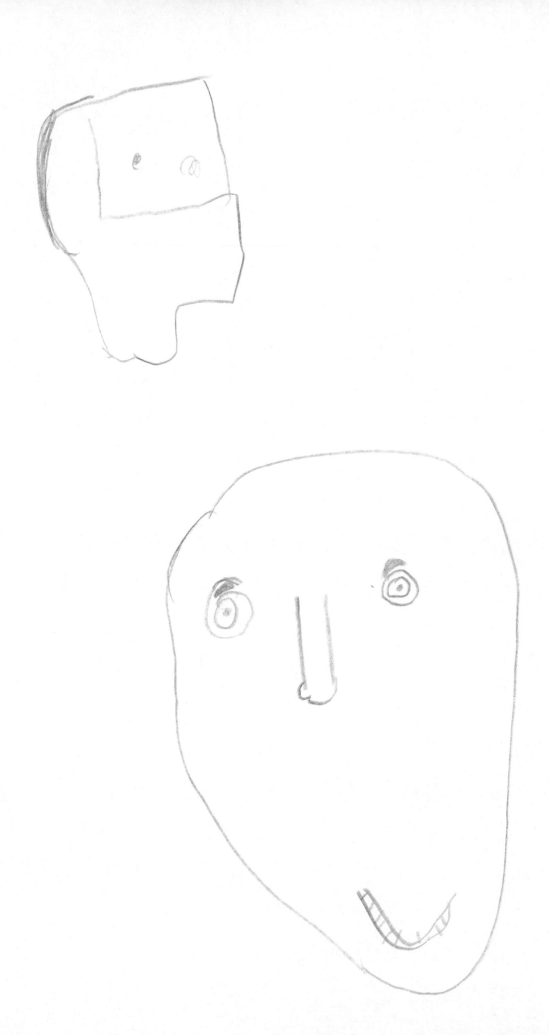

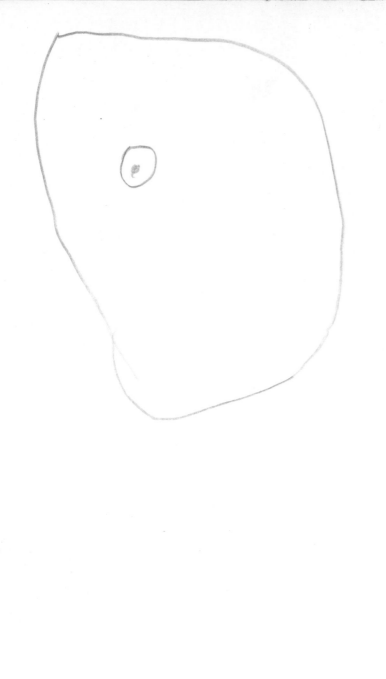